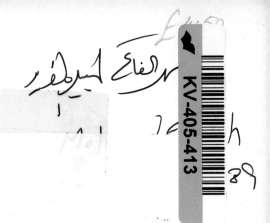

KV-405-413

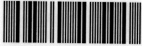

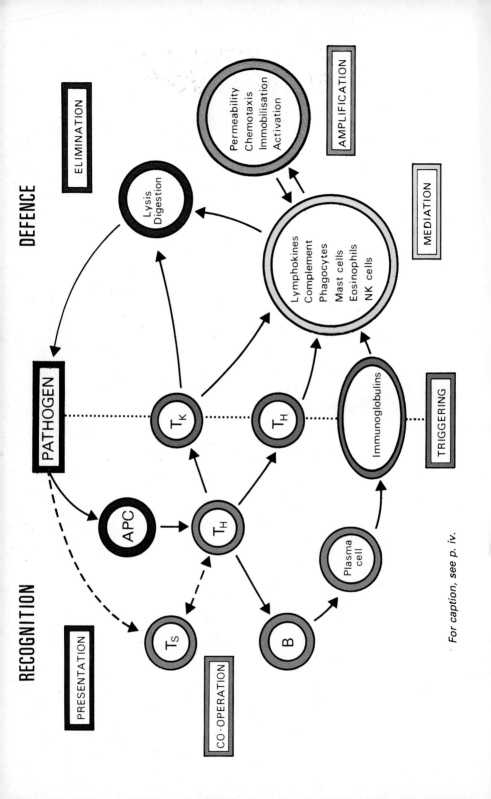

For caption, see p. iv.

# LECTURE NOTES ON
# IMMUNOLOGY

## W. G. REEVES

MB BS BSc FRCP FRCPath

*Professor of Immunology*
*University Hospital*
*Queen's Medical Centre*
*Nottingham*

## BLACKWELL SCIENTIFIC PUBLICATIONS

OXFORD LONDON EDINBURGH

BOSTON PALO ALTO MELBOURNE

© 1987 by
Blackwell Scientific Publications
Editorial Offices:
Osney Mead, Oxford OX2 OEL
  (*Orders*: Tel. 0865 240201)
8 John Street, London WC1N 2ES
23 Ainslie Place, Edinburgh EH3 6AJ
52 Beacon Street, Boston
  Massachusetts 02108, USA
667 Lytton Avenue, Palo Alto
  California 94301, USA
107 Barry Street, Carlton
  Victoria 3053, Australia

First published 1987

Set by Setrite Typesetters Ltd
Hong Kong
Printed and bound
in Great Britain

DISTRIBUTORS

USA
  Year Book Medical Publishers
  35 East Wacker Drive
  Chicago, Illinois 60601
  (*Orders*: Tel. 312 726−9733)

Canada
  The C.V. Mosby Company
  5240 Finch Avenue East,
  Scarborough, Ontario
  (*Orders*: Tel. 416−298−1588)

Australia
  Blackwell Scientific Publications
  (Australia) Pty Ltd
  107 Barry Street
  Carlton, Victoria 3053
  (*Orders*: Tel. (03) 347 0300)

British Library
Cataloguing in Publication Data

Reeves, W.G.
  Lecture notes on immunology.
  1. Immunology
  I. Title
  574.2′9     QR181
  ISBN 0−632−00776−1

*Frontispiece* (see p. ii): **A BIRD'S-EYE VIEW OF THE IMMUNE SYSTEM.**
**APC**—antigen presenting cell; $T_s$, $T_h$ and $T_k$—lymphocytes with suppressor, helper
and killer activities, respectively; **B**—B lymphocyte; **NK** cells—Natural Killer cells.
[This summary diagram is introduced in Chapter 1 prior to more detailed description
of its component parts in the chapters which follow.]

# Contents

# Preface

The undergraduate student meeting immunology during a busy medical or biological sciences curriculum or the qualified doctor attempting to get to grips with the subject for specialist training is often daunted by what appears to be an opaque wall of mystifying jargon surrounding a mass of intricate information. The aim of *Lecture Notes on Immunology* is to provide a concise statement covering the basic facts and concepts that are essential for a first understanding of the subject and its relevance to medicine and allied disciplines. Nomenclature has been simplified and appropriately defined and the major principles introduced in a biological setting. Figures and tables are used to summarise or highlight important information and key words are emphasised in the text in bold type. Brief but carefully selected lists of further reading are presented at the end of each chapter.

This text is based on the teaching modules developed in the Nottingham Medical School which have been designed to provide sufficient grounding to enable students to comprehend and utilise developments in immunology in their practice of medicine. Students often feel more comfortable with the detail when they have glimpsed the whole and for this reason the initial chapter outlines the salient features of immunity culminating in the 'bird's-eye view of the immune system' presented as Fig. 1.7 and the frontispiece. Chapters 2 to 9 then review the component parts which mediate recognition and defence. Chapters 10 to 15 cover the major areas of immunopathology, i.e. allergy, the pathology of infectious disease and autoimmunity; mechanisms and examples of immunological tissue damage; immunodeficiency and lympho-proliferative disease and conclude with chapters on transplantation and HLA and disease.

Many people have contributed, consciously or unconsciously, to the style and structure of this book and it is a pleasure to acknowledge the tutorial influence of Sydney Cohen, Peter Lachmann and John Holborow at different stages of my career. Several past and present members of my department in Nottingham have assisted in the development of our teaching programmes and Andrew Campbell, Ian Deverill, Graham Leslie, Denis Marriott, Richard Powell and Tim Wallington deserve special mention. I am also grateful to Ken MacLennan for assistance with the section on lymphomas. Many of my thoughts have been stimulated by the, often penetrating, questions of first year students as well as the more clinically informed enquiries of medical graduates and I hope that this text will assist the questioning process.

I am indebted to Sally Azadehdel who transformed my free-hand sketches into respectable figures and Joan Bennett who gave the manuscript her meticulous attention at all stages. Liffy, Sophie and Oliver Reeves supported in many ways throughout its gestation.

# IMMUNITY AND
# THE IMMUNE SYSTEM

# Chapter 1
# The nature of immunity

Infectious diseases, frequently compounded by malnutrition, are still the major cause of illness and death throughout the world. In developed countries, however, the situation has changed dramatically. In Britain, eighteenth century Bills of Mortality listed cholera, diphtheria, smallpox, tetanus and typhoid as major causes of death whereas today the annual mortality statistics emphasise the importance of cardiovascular disease and cancer. The balance has shifted so much that a series of deaths from a particular infectious disease is likely to precipitate the setting up of a committee of enquiry. These changes have been brought about by the introduction of successful immunisation programmes in conjunction with chemotherapy and various public health measures. The key role of the immune system in defence against pathogens of many kinds has recently received dramatic emphasis with the rapid spread of the acquired immunodeficiency syndrome (AIDS). Allergic hypersensitivity and auto-immunity are also recognised as disturbances of immunity which cause many other kinds of disease, e.g. asthma and glomerulonephritis. However, manipulation of the immune system is of increasing importance in the treatment of disease and in organ transplantation.

This all began with the centuries-old knowledge that an individual who had recovered from a life-threatening infection, e.g. plague could subsequently nurse another affected individual without fear of contracting the disease again. He or she had become **immune**. The term **immunity** was originally used to indicate exemption from taxes and this meaning still exists in the term 'diplomatic immunity'. The sequence of events that led to the global eradication of smallpox in 1980 spans more than two centuries and demonstrates vividly the way in which the immune response can be modified to render a previously life-threatening pathogen ineffective in causing disease.

## Variolation and vaccination

It is estimated that over 50 million people died of smallpox in eighteenth century Europe. In 1712, a duke's daughter from Nottinghamshire, Lady Mary Pierrepont, eloped with a diplomat, Edward Wortley-Montagu, and later travelled with him when he became British Ambassador to Turkey. She wrote from Constantinople in 1717 concerning the local habit of preventing smallpox by inoculating material obtained from smallpox crusts. She introduced it into England with Royal patronage following initial experiments on condemned criminals and orphaned children. However, this procedure was not without risk of causing smallpox (variola) itself and the high morbidity and mortality associated with it made others look for less dangerous and more effective ways of controlling the disease.

Edward Jenner — a Gloucestershire family doctor — made the important observation that dairymaids, who frequently contracted cowpox (an infection of the hands acquired during milking), were remarkably resistant to smallpox and did not develop the disfigured pock-marked faces of those that had had smallpox infection. Hence the rhyme:

> *'Where are you going to, my pretty maid?'*
> *'I'm going a-milking, sir', she said.*
> *'What is your fortune, my pretty maid?'*
> *'My face is my fortune, sir', she said.*

Edward Jenner had suffered painfully from variolation performed when he was eight years old. The increasing spread of smallpox throughout the population led him to develop the alternative technique of vaccination. This was first performed in 1796 when he inoculated material obtained from cowpox pustules into the arm of a healthy boy. He was subsequently able to inoculate him with smallpox more than 20 times without any untoward effect. This courageous experiment aroused much criticism but Jenner offered his new preventative treatment to all who sought it and performed many of his vaccinations in a thatched hut — which became known as the Temple of Vaccinia — in the grounds of his house at Berkeley. Recently, these buildings have been restored and contain a Jenner Museum and Conference Centre.*

Many other forms of immunisation have followed from this work and one of the current goals of the World Health Organisation's Tropical Disease Programme is to identify immunological ways of controlling and, hopefully, eliminating other major infec-

---

* Further information can be obtained from the Custodian, The Chantry, Church Lane, High Street, Berkeley, Gloucestershire GL13 9BH, UK.

tions, e.g. malaria (against which vector control has largely failed and chemotherapy is becoming less effective).

Several other kinds of immunological manipulation have proved to be of therapeutic benefit, e.g. the administration of specific antibody in the prevention of rhesus haemolytic disease of the newborn. The advent of monoclonal antibodies of many different specificities offers promise for targeting therapeutic agents to tissues and tumours as well as many diagnostic applications. Experimental work has shown that the administration of antigen or antibody can be used to turn off specific immune responses — a situation known as immunological tolerance or enhancement. Such a development would be of particular value for clinical transplantation and the treatment of many immunological and metabolic disorders.

## Cardinal features of immune responses

An individual who is immune to smallpox will not be protected against diphtheria unless he has also met the *Corynebacterium diphtheriae* on a previous occasion. This illustrates the **specificity** of the immune response. The immune response can detect remarkably small chemical differences between foreign materials, e.g. subtly differing strains of influenza virus, minor substitutions of a benzene ring, and the difference between dextro and laevo isomers. Were it not for the fact that cowpox and smallpox viruses share important antigens, the experiments of Edward Jenner would have been a dismal failure (although it is unlikely that he would have attempted them without the evidence of the milkmaids). Another feature of immune responses is the **memory** that develops for previous experiences of foreign material — a characteristic which enables immunisation to be of clinical value. This altered reactivity may last for the entire life-span of the individual.

The ability of an organism to respond more rapidly and to a greater degree when confronted with the same antigen on a second occasion is termed **amplification** and is illustrated in Fig. 1.1. This

**Table 1.1** Cardinal features of the immune response.

| |
|---|
| Specificity |
| Memory |
| Amplification |
| Self-discrimination |

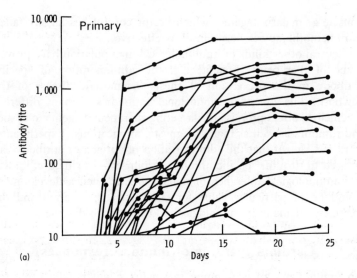

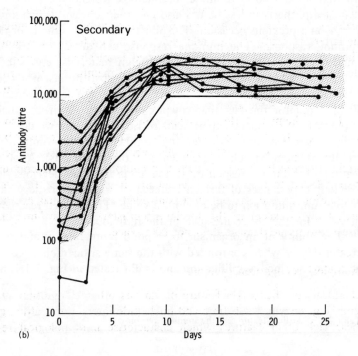

**Fig. 1.1** Primary and secondary antibody responses following intravenous injection of bacteriophage φX174 used as a test antigen in man. Data kindly provided by Drs Peacock and Verrier Jones.

compares the speed and magnitude of the human response to an antigen which the subjects had not previously encountered (bacteriophage φX174). In the first or **primary** response there is a delay of at least 10 days before the antibody level in the circulation reaches its maximum and this level shows considerable variation between individuals, few of whom exceed a titre* of 1000. In the **secondary** response all individuals respond maximally within 10 days and in all cases the levels attained are of a titre of 10 000 or more. As discussed below, the outcome of an acute infection is often a close race between the activities of the replicating pathogen and the adaptive immune response and it is for this reason that prior exposure, e.g. to a vaccine, can give the host a considerable head start.

Another important feature of immune responses is **self-discrimination**, which is illustrated in Fig. 1.2. In this experiment nine split-skin grafts are placed on the abdomen of a guinea pig. Eight days after grafting four of them appear healthy whereas the other five have become discoloured. At 16 days the former have healed well and are beginning to fill the remaining defect whereas the latter are being rejected and will soon slough from the wound. The four successful grafts were obtained from another animal of identical genetic composition (i.e. another member of the same inbred strain). The five rejected grafts came from an unrelated member of the same species.

These chemical differences are relatively minor and demonstrate not only the recognition ability of the immune system but also the efficient way in which it fails to react against tissue of 'self' origin. Previously, it was thought that components of the immune system failed to recognise self at all but it is now clear that self recognition does occur but in a controlled and regulated manner such that — except in the special circumstance of auto-immune disease — tissue damage does not take place.

## Biological recognition systems

Chemical specificity is a feature of various other recognition systems, e.g. enzyme–substrate and nucleotide interactions, although these lack other features which characterise immunological res-

---

* The *titre* is the reciprocal of the weakest dilution of serum at which antibody can still be detected.

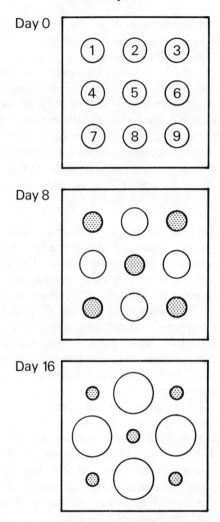

**Fig. 1.2** Discrimination between self and non-self illustrated by skin grafting in the guinea pig. Grafts 2, 4, 6 and 8 were of 'self' type; the others were from an unrelated animal.

ponses. It is likely that the recognition component of immune responses has developed from a more basic cellular attribute by which cells are able to recognise each other. Evidence for complementary cell surface interactions has come from several different areas of biological research, e.g. the cellular reaggregation of multicellular invertebrate organisms, e.g. sponges and slime moulds; the processes whereby cells differentially associate during embryogenesis; the way in which synaptic connections are established in the nervous system; and the recognition events involved in pollination and fertilisation. Analogy with these other systems suggests that recognition of self is a primary requirement in phylogeny which, in complex mammalian organisms, has developed into a more sophisticated arrangement whereby reactions to self and non-self have been separately harnessed. Antigens and their recognition are discussed in more detail in Chapter 2.

## Recognition and defence: a minimal model

Before considering the complexity of what is known it is useful to conjecture how one might design an immune system in order to protect the host organism and display the characteristic features already described. Clearly, the two important biological events are **recognition** of the target pathogen and effective **defence** against it. A major consideration is how many recognition specificities are required and how many kinds of defence, i.e. methods of pathogen destruction, are necessary. The next question to be decided is whether the units that recognise and the units that defend should be combined together or whether a division of labour is preferable in which recognition units and defence units operate as separate entities. Using the military analogy, the former is equivalent to hand-to-hand fighting and the latter comparable to artillery support invoked by those in the front line. These rival possibilities are set out Lego-style in Fig. 1.3.

Whichever aggressive modality is preferred, it is necessary to plan for rapid adaptation — quantitatively either upwards or downwards — depending on the circumstances. This has implications for the supply of materials and whether the number of recognition and defence units need to be increased in equal proportion. Recognition units, at least, will need to circulate to all parts of the host organism which may be under threat and this will have implications for the size of unit that can permeate into extravascular sites. It is likely that defence units will require greater chemical complexity than those involved in recognition and this has implications for the economy of supplies.

If recognition and defence units occur as separate entities (Fig. 1.3b) then a means has to be developed whereby the latter can be specifically recruited to the site where recognition units have de-

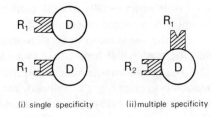

(a) COMBINED RECOGNITION AND DEFENCE UNITS

(i) single specificity     (ii) multiple specificity

(b) RECOGNITION AND DEFENCE AS SEPARATE ENTITIES

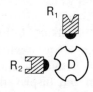

(i) single kind of activator

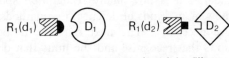

(ii) different kinds of activator ($d_1$, $d_2$) for different defence units ($D_1$, $D_2$)

**Fig. 1.3** Possible arrangements of recognition (R) and defence (D) units to deal with a pathogenic invader. See text.

tected their target and an arrangement has to be devised for defence units to be activated only when their complementary recognition unit has recognised its target. Theoretically, the latter could be achieved either by a conformational change developing in the recognition unit (comparable to the steric changes involved in enzyme–substrate interactions) or, alternatively, one could envisage a requirement whereby defence units were only triggered when several of their complementary recognition units become aggregated together on a specific target. It would also be important for the toxic inflammatory products of defence units to be very well contained prior to release or only to be synthesised when the unit has become activated. It also might be necessary for inhibitory factors to be present which can limit the scale of the toxic effect of destructive molecules released in proximity to the specific target. If several biologically different kinds of destructive activity are required then different classes of activator will need to be present within the repertoire of recognition units (Fig. 1.3 b(ii)).

As the details of the immune system are reviewed in the succeeding chapters, the reader will realise that each of these different solutions to the basic requirement are found in real life, e.g. killer T cells are combined recognition and defence units each bearing a single specificity (as a(i)) whereas NK cells are combined recognition and defence units which are much less specific in their target recognition. Immunoglobulins contain a large repertoire of recognition units many of which can activate identical defence units, e.g. complement (as b(i)), but which have also undergone specialisation with the development of different classes of activator for different effector systems, e.g. complement vs. phagocytes vs. mast cells (as in b(ii)). In summary, the immune system seems to have discovered most ways of doing things and, as will be seen later, much of its complexity undoubtedly arises from the very extensive and varied demands made upon it.

## Immunological recognition

The first clue to the identity of immunological recognition units derived from studies performed by Paul Ehrlich and his colleagues in the 1890s on factors present in serum which could transfer a state of immunity to a non-immune animal or person. Most of this work focused on toxin-producing organisms, e.g. diphtheria, cholera and tetanus. It was demonstrated that serum factors or 'antitoxins' which developed in the serum of an immune individual were specific for each particular infection. This led Ehrlich to develop his 'side-chain' or receptor hypothesis of immunity in which the numbers of side-chains or receptors available to recognise a foreign specificity could increase in response to an infective stimulus and might possess a separate ability to 'take to itself ferment-like material'. Clearly, he was favouring the possibility outlined in Fig. 1.3 b(i). When protein electrophoresis was introduced in the 1930s it was possible to localise these specific factors or **antibodies** to the $\gamma$-globulin fraction and detailed chemical studies performed by Porter and Edelman culminated in the elucidation of the four-chain structure of these bifunctional **immunoglobulin** molecules in the early 1960s. The structure and function of immunoglobulins are considered in detail in Chapter 5. The plasma cell was identified as the source of serum immunoglobulins in 1948 but their static behaviour and brief lifespan made it unlikely that they were the cells which made first contact with those element of foreign materials which could generate an antibody response, i.e. **antigens.**

Chase and his colleagues had observed that the immunological reaction induced by the cutaneous application of certain chemicals — known as contact or delayed hypersensitivity — could be transferred from one animal to another by the infusion of lymphoid cells. However, Gowans took advantage of the natural process whereby **lymphocytes** are separated from the other white cells of the blood to form the sole cellular constituent of lymph. He found that animals depleted of lymphocytes by thoracic duct drainage lost their ability to respond to antigens to which they had previously been immunised and also failed to reject foreign grafts. Immunological responsiveness was restored when their lymphocytes were returned to them by intravenous infusion. It was this work (also in the early 1960s) that caused the lymphocyte to be recognised as the pre-eminent **immunocompetent cell**. However, the link between the freely circulating lymphocyte and the immunoglobulin-producing plasma cell was not established until the 1970s.

## T and B lymphocytes

Peripheral blood lymphocytes are indistinguishable from each other when examined using traditional Leishman or Giemsa stains and it was only when attempts were made to detect the presence of the immunoglobulin recognition units within their surface that a major distinction could be drawn. Using the technique of immunofluorescence it was discovered that about 15 per cent of circulating lymphocytes possessed **surface immunoglobulin**. Other work indicated that it was this subset of lymphocytes which transformed into the immunoglobulin-secreting plasma cell following contact with specific antigen. Experiments performed in the chicken showed that these lymphocytes required a period of differentiation in a gut-associated lymphoid organ known as the Bursa of Fabricius — and for this reason these cells became designated **B lymphocytes** (Fig. 1.4). The other major subset of lymphocytes responded to antigen independently of antibody, and was found to contain a surface glycoprotein with high affinity for a component of the surface of sheep red blood cells. The formation of sheep red blood cell 'rosettes' when the two cell types were mixed together provided a useful marker for this lymphocyte subset. It was also demonstrated

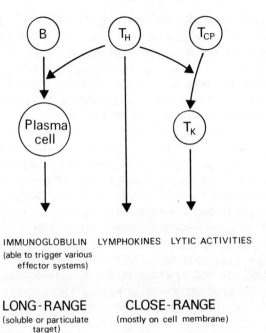

IMMUNOGLOBULIN   LYMPHOKINES   LYTIC ACTIVITIES
(able to trigger various
effector systems)

LONG-RANGE          CLOSE-RANGE
(soluble or particulate    (mostly on cell membrane)
target)

**Fig. 1.4** The biological roles of lymphocyte subpopulations.

that these cells required a period of differentiation in the **thymus** and this gave rise to the designation **T lymphocytes**.

The immunoglobulin on the surface of B cells is the specific antigen receptor which, when the B cell transforms into a plasma cell, is secreted as a soluble product capable of interaction with the antigen at a distance from the cell in which it was produced. The nature of the antigen receptor on T cells is still a subject of active research and debate although considerable advances have taken place in the last few years. Although it belongs to the same family of surface recognition molecules as immunoglobulins and histocompatibility glycoproteins, it possesses significant differences and recognises antigen in a different way. Immunoglobulins are designed to interact with pathogens (and parts thereof) which are not intimately associated with cells of the host organism. The T cell receptor, however, is designed so that successful interaction only takes place when antigen is recognised in close association with molecules representative of self cell membranes. These characteristics are reviewed in Chapters 3 and 4.

Further specialisation is evident within both B and T lympho-cyte populations, the main subsets of the latter being the helper T cell and the T cells which mediate killer or suppressor activities. The **helper T cell** occupies the central position in immunity, with-out which the B cell cannot differentiate into the immunoglobulin-secreting plasma cell and without which the **killer T cell** does not become activated from a cytotoxic precursor ($T_{cp}$) (Fig. 1.4). Each of these lymphocyte subpopulations can be identified by various surface markers and although the surface characteristics of suppres-sor T cells and killer T cells usually coincide it is still not clear how these two rather different functions are executed.

Most human studies, of necessity, focus on lymphocytes in the circulation rather than in lymphoid tissues but it is in the latter that the very large majority of lymphocytes reside (Fig. 1.5). Lympho-cytes develop in **primary lymphoid organs**, consisting of bone marrow and thymus, in the adult. Lymphocytes circulate through **lymph nodes**, the white pulp of the **spleen** and **mucosa-associated lymphoid tissue** (**MALT**): these locations are referred to as **se-**

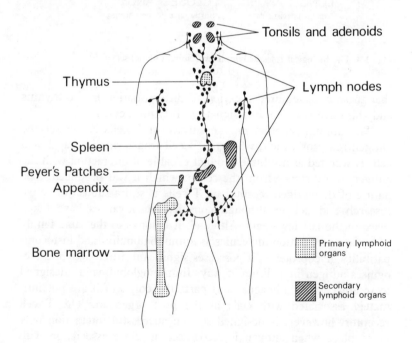

**Fig. 1.5** Distribution of primary and secondary lymphoid organs in man.

**condary lymphoid organs**. The total weight of these various lymphoid components can exceed that of the liver. It is at these various sites that the different varieties of lymphocyte come into intimate contact with each other and with specialised antigen-presenting cells. Lymphocytes and lymphoid organs are discussed more fully in Chapter 3.

## Immunological defence

Early observations indicated that additional components, e.g. complement (discovered by Jules Bordet) and phagocytes (first identified by Elie Metchnikoff), were necessary for the successful elimination of pathogens. Different kinds of defence unit do require their own triggering mechanism (as in Fig. 1.3 b(ii)) and Table 1.2 lists the major defence or effector systems, the recognition units which trigger them and their means of pathogen lysis. They have considerable inflammatory potential and each system has its own internal control mechanisms to reduce the possibility of inappropriate activation and damage to host tissues. The details of these various systems are reviewed in Chapters 6—9. In each case, the terminal act of pathogen destruction is preceded by a series of amplifying events that serve to recruit and harness all the relevant cells and molecules required to achieve the *coup de grâce* by extracellular lysis or intracellular digestion. These amplifying events can be divided into four categories: a local increase in vascular **permeability**, chemical attraction of inflammatory cells, i.e. **chemotaxis, immobilisation** of cells at the site of inflammation, and **activation** of the relevant cells and molecules to liberate their lytic products (Fig. 1.6).

**Table 1.2** Effector systems, their triggers and means of lysis.

| System | Trigger | Lysis |
|---|---|---|
| Complement | IgG, IgM, IgA | extracellular |
| Neutrophils | IgG, IgA | intracellular |
| Macrophages | IgG, IgE | intracellular |
| Mast cells | IgE | — |
| Eosinophils | IgG, IgE | extracellular |
| NK/LGL cells | ? | extracellular |
| Lymphokines | T cell receptor | extracellular |

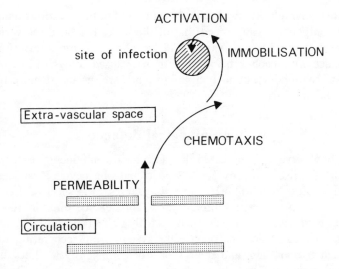

**Fig. 1.6** Amplifying events involved in the local recruitment of inflammatory cells and molecules from the circulation into an extravascular site of infection.

## A bird's-eye view

The complexities of the immune system often seem rather daunting to the novice although students usually find the necessary detail more manageable when they can see how the individual parts fit together into a coherent whole. Figure 1.7 gives a diagrammatic overview of the immune system incorporating the individual components to which reference has already been made and emphasises the important distinction between those parts of the immune system which specifically recognise the chemical nature of the pathogen and those components which are triggered to act non-specifically and effect its inflammatory destruction.

The abundance of means by which recognition and defence can be achieved is surprising and begs the question of why so many alternative pathways have developed during evolution. However, there are similarities as well as differences and the various forms of (a) recognition units, (b) effector systems and (c) lytic processes show considerable homology and may have developed as genetic variants of common ancestral systems.

The stimulus for such diversification arises from the enormous task with which the immune system is confronted, i.e. the constant

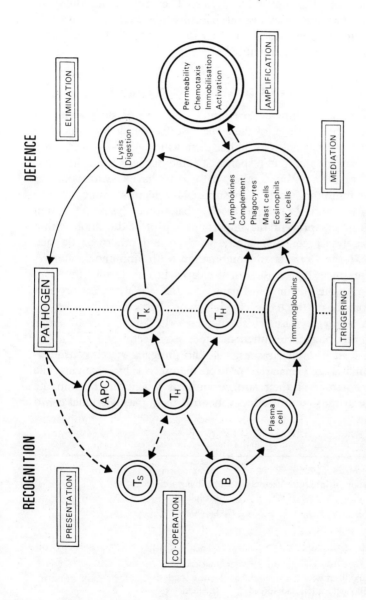

**Fig. 1.7 A bird's-eye view of the immune system.** The recognition compartment concerns the events by which a pathogen is recognised and presented to the specifically reacting components culminating in the production of cells and molecules able to trigger the various non-specific mediator systems by which effective defence is mounted. These processes are discussed further in the text. APC — antigen presenting cell; $T_s$, $T_h$ and $T_k$ — T lymphocytes with suppressor, helper and killer activities, respectively; B — B lymphocyte; NK cells — Natural Killer cells. (See also colour frontispiece.)

threat to the survival of the host from a universe of pathogenic organisms ranging from the smallest viruses to metazoan parasites with their often complex life cycles. The remarkable ability of successful parasites to evolve mechanisms by which they can evade the immune response adds a further dimension which is currently receiving considerable attention.

## Evasion of the immune response

Pneumococci are difficult to eliminate because of their ability to produce large quantities of their major surface antigen — pneumococcal polysaccharide — in soluble form which acts as a 'decoy' and preoccupies the immune response at some distance from the replicating organism. Many other pathogens have been found to produce inhibitory or immunosuppressive factors: some such as *Toxoplasma* and *Legionella* block phagosome–lysosome fusion whereas others prevent the important step of acidification within the phagolysosome. Gonococci, which would otherwise be susceptible to the effects of combination with immunoglobulin A (IgA), produce a protease which cleaves IgA molecules into Fab and Fc portions (defined in Chapter 5). *Bordetella pertussis* protects itself from the destructive events following phagocytosis by releasing its own adenyl cyclase which increases the level of cyclic AMP and inhibits phagocyte function.

Other successful parasites, e.g. the protozoa which cause trypanosomiasis and malaria, protect themselves by changing the chemical nature of their surface antigens whenever the immune response begins to deal effectively with them. Schistosomes avoid

**Table 1.3** Mechanisms of evasion of the immune response.

| | |
|---|---|
| Release of soluble antigen | pneumococci |
| Production of inhibitory factors | staphylococci |
| | toxoplasmosis |
| | gonococci |
| | *B. pertussis* |
| | *Legionella* |
| Antigenic variation | trypanosomiasis |
| | malaria |
| Antigenic disguise | schistosomiasis |
| Intracellular location and spread | tuberculosis |
| | leishmaniasis |
| | budding viruses |

**Table 1.4** Categories of immunopathological disorder.

Allergy or hypersensitivity
Auto-immunity
Lympho-proliferative disease
Immunodeficiency

attention by a process of antigenic disguise in which they coat themselves with host blood group glycoproteins. A number of other pathogens, e.g. mycobacteria, *Leishmania* and budding viruses, gain a degree of protection by their location within host cells.

## The host : pathogen interface

The outcome of a particular infection depends on many factors which govern the ability of the pathogen to invade, evade and damage the host and the ability of the immune response to recognise, trigger, amplify and destroy the pathogen. Any weakening of the pathogen (often referred to as attenuation) or strengthening of the specific immune response against it (e.g. by immunisation) will favour the success of the immune response whereas successful means of evasion displayed by the parasite or the development of immunodeficiency (be it inherited or acquired) will tip the scales in favour of the pathogen. This interrelationship has been spoken of as 'a game of chess played over millions of years'.

It is thus not surprising that the outcome for the host is often 'survival at a price' and that damage to host tissues is a common finding during the course of most infectious diseases — a situation referred to as **hypersensitivity** or **allergy**. Furthermore, the development of **auto-immunity** is not uncommon during infection and

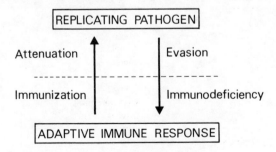

**Fig. 1.8** The host : pathogen interface and factors which affect it.

H002 3645

the chronicity of these reactions may be related to the difficulties involved in eliminating certain pathogens from host cells. Some pathogens are also able to initiate various forms of **lympho-proliferative disease** and can cause **immunodeficiency** (Table 1.4). **Immunopathology** is comprised of these various deviations from the ideal, many examples of which are found in human disease.

# Further reading

Cox F.E.G. ed. (1982) *Modern Parasitology.* Blackwell Scientific Publications, Oxford.

Greaves M.F. (1975) *Cellular Recognition.* Chapman & Hall, London.

Herbert W.J., Wilkinson P.C. & Stott D.I. eds (1985) *Dictionary of Immunology*, 3rd edn. Blackwell Scientific Publications, Oxford.

Holborow E.J. & Reeves W.G. eds (1983) *Immunology in Medicine: a Comprehensive Guide to Clinical Immunology*, 2nd edn. Grune & Stratton, London.

Mims C.A. (1982) *The Pathogenesis of Infectious Disease*, 2nd edn. Academic Press, London.

O'Grady F. & Smith H. eds (1981) *Microbial Perturbation of Host Defences.* Academic Press, London.

Rains A.J.H. (1974) *Edward Jenner and Vaccination.* Priory Press, London.

# Chapter 2
# Antigens and antigen recognition

Most forms of biological material can be recognised by the immune system and those constituents that can generate an immune response are referred to as **antigens** or **immunogens**. Macromolecular proteins are the most potent but polysaccharides, glycoproteins, synthetic polypeptides and synthetic polymers can also be immunogenic. Lipids and nucleic acids are not usually immunogenic unless conjugated to a protein moiety and nucleoproteins readily induce antibodies reactive with nucleic acids.

## Terminology

A variety of terms has been used to describe the recognisable components of antigenic material (Table 2.1). The smallest of these is known as an antigenic **determinant, epitope** or **hapten**, and represents the discrete configuration that interacts with the combining site of an antibody molecule. Studies using defined antigens indicate that its size is equivalent to a tetrapeptide or hexasaccharide. Material of this size can complex with appropriately specific antibody molecules present in body fluids or on the surface of B lymphocytes. It is not, however, able to initiate an immune response. For this to occur, B lymphocytes require help from appropriately stimulated T lymphocytes. The minimum requirement for the combined stimulation of T and B cells is the presentation of a larger molecule in which the epitope or hapten is conjugated to a T cell-stimulating **carrier** component (see Fig. 2.1). This complete antigen is sometimes referred to as a **hapten−carrier** complex although a determinant that acts as hapten in one response may well act as carrier in another. The terms **immunogen** or **antigen** are more commonly used as synonyms for the hapten−carrier complex.

**Table 2.1** Terms used to describe structures recognised by the immune system.

| Antigen | = | immunogen | = | hapten−carrier complex |
|---|---|---|---|---|
| Determinant | = | epitope | = | hapten |
| Tolerogen | | | | |

*Chapter 2*

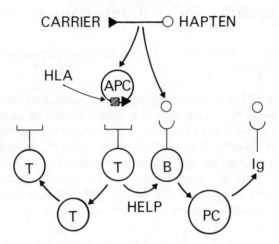

**Fig. 2.1** The recognition of antigens by T and B lymphocytes. APC = antigen-presenting cell, HLA = HLA glycoprotein, Ig = immunoglobulin and PC = plasma cell. The way in which T cells help B cells is discussed in the text.

The requirement for covalent linkage between hapten and carrier determinants has been demonstrated experimentally, the optimum size of the antigen bridge being of the order of $50 \times 10^{-10}$m. However, it is not yet clear whether the bridge mediates direct contact between T and B lymphocytes or whether it interacts with antigen-specific soluble factors derived from these cells.

Some molecules, e.g. bacterial polysaccharides and some polymerised proteins, have a structure which consists of a series of repeating subunits. These show very little requirement for T cell help and induce antibody responses which are mostly of IgM class and with little or no immunological memory. These materials are often referred to as T-independent antigens although their distinction from the more widespread T-dependent antigens is likely to be quantitative rather than qualitative in nature.

Some materials, e.g. aggregate-free proteins administered in soluble form can induce a specific immunological response of a negative kind known as immunological **tolerance**. Exposure to a **tolerogen** is not followed by a detectable response but causes the animal to become specifically unresponsive to subsequent challenge with a normally immunogenic form of the same material.

The T and B lymphocytes stimulated in a particular immune

response each bear receptors which are chemically specific for determinants on the stimulating antigen. Mammalian organisms are capable of responding to many different kinds of chemical determinant and it has been estimated that there is of the order of $10^7$ varieties of lymphocyte each with a different kind of antigen-specific receptor. In the case of B lymphocytes this receptor is immunoglobulin and is released into the circulation in significant quantities by the plasma cells which differentiate from them. The antigen-combining sites of immunoglobulin molecules show considerable chemical variation (see Chapter 5) and the chemical individuality of a particular molecule is often referred to as the **idiotype**.

The T lymphocyte receptor shows some overall similarity with immunoglobulin molecules but has other interesting differences. The major functional difference is that T helper cells are only activated when antigen is presented in close association with histocompatibility glycoproteins (belonging to the HLA system — see Chapter 4) on the surface of antigen-presenting cells (Fig. 2.1). This is known as **dual recognition** and it has been shown in experimental systems that T cells are only stimulated by antigen in association with HLA proteins of 'self' type. T helper cells are not only able to help or induce B cells to transform into plasma cells but also have an inducer function with respect to other T cells, e.g. T killer cells, and expand the pool of T helper cells.

## Factors governing immunogenicity

Table 2.2 lists the factors of major importance. Smaller molecules are less immunogenic and the smaller the molecule the greater is the individual variation in response. The threshold for immunogenicity varies but is of the order of 1500 MW. Charged residues

**Table 2.2** Factors governing immunogenicity.

| Antigen | size |
| --- | --- |
| | charge |
| | chemical nature |
| | foreignness |
| | dose |
| | frequency |
| | route |
| Recipient | genes |
| | nutrition |

tend to contribute to the specificity of immunogens as they are usually expressed on the hydrophilic surface of the molecule but uncharged molecules such as dextrans can be immunogenic. Structural complexity and the degree of foreignness of a molecule (compared to that possessed by the host animal) are important factors and molecules which are not normally immunogenic can become so when denatured or aggregated. Every antigen has an optimum dose for immunogenicity and in experimental systems doses significantly lower or higher than the optimum can induce 'low zone' or 'high zone' tolerance, respectively. Intermittent immunisation usually produces a greater response than a period of continuous administration. Experimentally, the immune response is usually increased by mixing the antigen with a powerful adjuvant, e.g. a mycobacterial extract, which intensifies the inflammatory response nonspecifically.

The route of immunisation is also of importance: oral administration can induce tolerance to subsequent challenge via the usually immunogenic parenteral route (the Schulzberger–Chase phenomenon). Variations on the part of the host can also affect the outcome. Malnutrition or metabolic disturbance (as in uncontrolled diabetes) impairs immune responses. Significant genetic effects can be observed when well-defined antigens of modest size are used, e.g. insulin, and this variation has been shown to associate with particular phenotypes of both the HLA and the immunoglobulin allotype (Gm) systems.

## Antigen-presenting cells (APC)

Antigenic material is only effective in inducing an immune response when it is processed and presented to specific clones of lymphocytes by antigen-presenting cells (APC) (sometimes called accessory cells). Soluble antigens that make direct contact with T or B cells are likely to induce specific unresponsiveness. Until relatively recently, peripheral blood monocytes and tissue **macrophages** were considered to be the major APC. Not only are they phagocytic but they also process antigenic material and express it on their surface in close association with class II HLA glycoproteins (see p. 46). It is now clear that other cells, e.g. follicular dendritic, interdigitating dendritic and Langerhans cells, are very effective at antigen presentation *in vivo* (see Table 2.3).

**Follicular dendritic cells** are present in germinal centres in lymphoid tissue (see Fig. 3.5) and retain antigen for long periods.

**Table 2.3**  Surface markers of antigen-presenting cells.

|  | Class II HLA glycoprotein | Fc receptor | C3 receptor |
| --- | --- | --- | --- |
| Classical macrophages | + | + | + |
| Follicular dendritic cells | − | + | + |
| Interdigitating dendritic cells | + | − | − |
| Langerhans cells | + | + | + |

There is good evidence that antigen in the form of immune complexes is preferentially taken up by these cells, which then interact with the B lymphocytes which surround them and expand the number of B memory cells for the antigen concerned. They, like classical macrophages, have receptors for the tail of immunoglobulin molecules (Fc receptors) and the third component of complement (C3 receptors) but lack class II HLA glycoproteins on their surface. In contrast, the **interdigitating dendritic cells** found diffusely throughout the paracortex of lymph nodes (Fig. 3.5) are exceptionally good at presenting antigens to T helper cells and express class II glycoproteins but lack Fc and C3 receptors. Both kinds of cell possess long finger-like processes which enable them to interact with large numbers of lymphocytes and both are non-phagocytic.

It seems probable that in the development of a mature immune response it is necessary for both kinds of antigen presentation to occur, i.e. via antibody-complexed antigen to expand the population of B memory cells within germinal centres as well as via HLA class II positive dendritic cells to stimulate T helper cells within the adjacent paracortex. This enables effective co-operation to take place between specific clones of T and B lymphocytes relevant to the individual immune response.

The **Langerhans cell** is present in the epidermis and possesses class II glycoproteins as well as Fc and C3 receptors. It is also very effective at antigen presentation and makes its way through the afferent lymph (where because of its distinctive appearance it has been referred to as 'veiled' or dendritic) to become the interdigitating cell of the paracortex. This cell is, like the classical macrophage, of bone marrow origin whereas follicular dendritic cells are not. The inset to Fig. 3.5 illustrates the sites in which the clonal expansion of specifically reactive T and B lymphocytes takes place in the lymph node. The differentiation and expansion of these clones of T and B lymphocytes are associated with the release of various soluble factors (see p. 40).

# T and B cell co-operation

Direct cell-to-cell contact is probably necessary for the successful interaction between antigen-presenting cells and T or B lymphocytes with release of the soluble factor **interleukin 1** being an additional requirement for triggering the helper T cell. Direct contact has often been considered necessary for effective co-operation between T and B lymphocytes and this may occur at an intermediate point in the lymph node or within the germinal centre itself (as small numbers of T helper cells have been identified within it). Alternatively, the appropriate signal for B cell differentiation into antibody-secreting plasma cells may be achieved by other soluble factors released from T cells which reach B cells within the germinal centre or as they migrate towards the medulla.

Recent work suggests that B cells themselves are also able to process and present antigen to T cells. If direct contact between these two cells is a common event then both antigen presentation and B cell triggering could occur in rapid succession. This, more streamlined, sequence of events is more likely to be of importance in the secondary immune response, in which specifically reactive cells of both types will be reasonably plentiful.

# Effects of antigen on lymphoid tissue

The arrival of antigen causes a number of dramatic changes in the local lymph node. There is a marked increase in blood supply associated with enlargement of post-capillary venules and opening of arteriovenous shunts. Large numbers of lymphocytes become trapped in the node and this phenomenon of cell shut-down is probably mediated by a combination of complement activation and prostaglandin release (e.g. $PGE_2$). Trapping is initially non-specific but antigen-reactive lymphocytes progressively accumulate and are no longer detectable in the efferent lymph. These changes cause considerable lymph node swelling.

A biphasic increase in lymphocyte output is detectable 2–4 days after the arrival of antigen: the first peak contains small resting lymphocytes non-specifically trapped during shut-down whereas the second peak contains blast cells which migrate to regions similar to those where they initially encountered antigen. These homing patterns are determined by structures on the surface of stimulated lymphocytes and the endothelial cells of the post-capillary venules which they traverse. Specific antibody is first detectable in the efferent lymph at around day 5.

# Further reading

Humphrey J.H. (1982) The fate of antigens. In Lachmann P.J. & Peters D.K. eds. *Clinical Aspects of Immunology*, 4th edn. Blackwell Scientific Publications, Oxford.

Feldman M., Katz D.R. & Sunshine G.H. (1984) RES–leukocyte interactions. In Reichard S.M. & Filkins J.P. eds. *The Reticuloendothelial System*, Vol. 7A. Plenum Press, New York.

Durum S.K., Schmidt J.A. & Oppenheim J.J. (1985) Interleukin 1: an immunological perspective. *Annual Review of Immunology*, 3, 263–87.

# Chapter 3
# Lymphocytes and lymphoid organs

Little was known about the function of lymphocytes until 30 years ago when experiments performed by Gowans demonstrated that the lymphocyte was the immunocompetent cell without which the immune system lost its ability to recognise and respond to antigen. He showed that rats depleted of their lymphocytes by continuous thoracic duct drainage failed to reject foreign grafts and lost the ability to develop delayed hypersensitivity reactions and antibody responses. Each of these activities could be restored by returning the lymphocytes intravenously.

Lymphocytes are derived from haemopoietic stem cells present, sequentially, in the yolk sac, liver and bone marrow. The primitive lymphoid cells which originate from bone marrow develop into two major populations of lymphocytes. Those that require a period of differentiation in the thymus are called **T cells**. In birds, B cells differentiate in a lymphoid component of the hindgut — the Bursa of Fabricius. Mammalian **B cells**, however, continue to differentiate without the need for a special micro-environment. Another major difference between these two populations of lymphocytes is that self-reactivity is rarely detected amongst the T cell population whereas B lymphocytes are not so restricted. This difference is due to events that take place in the thymus.

## The thymus

The epithelial component develops from the third and fourth pharyngeal pouches. The epithelial cells are soon joined by pre-T cells derived from bone marrow stem cells which become the rapidly dividing thymocytes of the cortex and interact with thymic macrophages and epithelial cells, both of which express histocompatibility proteins (class II HLA) on their surface. There is considerable proliferation and death of cortical thymocytes and it is likely that T cells with receptors for HLA proteins of self type are preferentially stimulated to proliferate and become eliminated whereas those T cells bearing receptors with low affinity for self antigens are allowed to mature and leave the thymus as functional T cells. Thymocytes are particularly responsive to interleukin 1 released by class II HLA-bearing accessory cells although the mechanism by which self-reactive T cells are eliminated is still unclear. The medulla is much less active and contains complex aggregates of epithelial cells — Hassall's corpuscles — the function of which is unknown. Some of the differentiative effects of the thymic environment have been reproduced using soluble extracts of thymic tissue, e.g. thymosin and thymopoietin.

A 'library' of molecules representative of self is thus exhibited in the developing thymus and self-reactivity is eliminated from the mature T cell population. A consequence of this is that surviving T cells with low affinity for self HLA proteins display a higher affinity for the HLA proteins present on other genetically non-identical members of the same species, i.e. they display allo-reactivity (see p. 43). This is in keeping with the fact that T lymphocytes are programmed by virtue of their surface receptors to recognise all foreign antigens in association with self HLA glycoproteins (see p. 32).

# T lymphocytes

T lymphocytes were first distinguished from B lymphocytes because of their lack of surface immunoglobulin (detectable by immunofluorescence) and their ability to form rosettes with sheep red blood cells. In recent years a number of other surface markers have been identified specific for T cells at various stages of their development (Fig. 3.1 and Table 3.1). Many of these have been discovered using monoclonal antibodies raised against T cells. The CD2 marker is identical with the membrane protein that binds sheep red blood cells and is present on all cells of the T cell series whereas CD3 is present on medullary thymocytes and all peripheral T cells and is associated with the T cell receptor for antigen.

## T cell subpopulations

A great deal of evidence points to the existence of functional and surface marker heterogeneity among T cells. The first observations showed that some T cells provided help for B lymphocytes by releasing growth factors, e.g. interleukin 2 and B cell growth factors, to enable them to differentiate into antibody secreting plasma cells. These have been termed **T helper** ($T_h$) cells. Another subset was shown to mediate cytotoxicity, e.g. against virus-infected or allo-

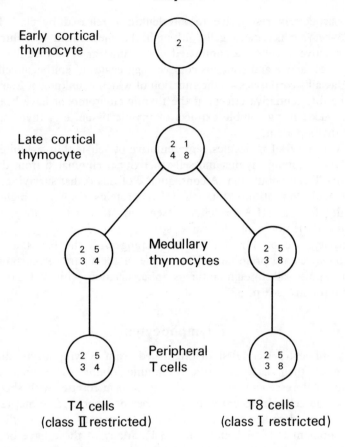

Early cortical
thymocyte

Late cortical
thymocyte

Medullary
thymocytes

Peripheral
T cells

T4 cells                          T8 cells
(class II restricted)        (class I restricted)

**Fig. 3.1** Stages of T cell differentiation using the CD nomenclature for surface markers. See Table 3.1 and text for further details.

geneic cells, and are called **T killer** ($T_k$) cells (Fig. 3.2). T helper cells also have a role in promoting the differentiation of $T_k$ cells from a cytotoxic precursor ($T_{cp}$) (as depicted in Fig. 1.4). Some T lymphocytes are able to suppress immune responses and have been designated $T_s$. Others are potent in releasing lymphokines which attract and activate other mononuclear cells, e.g. monocytes, and are prominent in delayed hypersensitivity reactions. These have been designated $T_{dh}$.

A number of monoclonal antibodies have been used to try and identify these functionally different T lymphocyte subsets. An international workshop has reviewed these various specificities and

**Table 3.1** Nomenclature for T cell markers.

| CD[a] | T[b] | Other | Positive cells |
|---|---|---|---|
| 1 | 6 | Leu[c]6 | Late cortical thymocytes |
| 2 | 11 | SRBC[d] | All cells of T lineage |
| 3 | 3 | Leu 4 | Medullary thymocytes and all peripheral T cells |
| 4 | 4 | Leu 3a | A subset of T cells |
| 5 | 1 | Leu 1 | Medullary thymocytes and all peripheral T cells |
| 8 | 8 | Leu 2 | A subset of T cells |
| 25 | – | T$_{ac}$ | IL-2 receptor on activated T cells |

[a]CD = cluster of differentiation defined by the First International Workshop on Human Leucocyte Differentiation Antigens (1982).
[b]T = Ortho (OKT) reagent specificities. [c]Leu = Becton-Dickinson reagent specificities. [d]SRBC = receptor for sheep red blood cell binding.

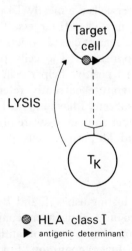

**Fig. 3.2** Dual recognition of antigen in association with class I HLA by the T8 positive killer cell.

produced a new nomenclature based on 'clusters of differentiation' (CD) by which each surface marker is defined (see Bernard *et al.* 1984). Some of these **CD markers** are listed in Table 3.1.

The pathway by which T cells differentiate and the CD markers present at each stage are set out in Fig. 3.1, from which it is seen that peripheral T cells consist of two phenotypically distinct populations of **T4** and **T8** cells, usually in the proportion of $c$. 65 per cent T4 to 35 per cent T8 although this bias is reversed in many immunological disorders. It had been thought for some time that the T4 marker identified the functional T helper cell (and probably $T_{dh}$, as well) whereas T8 identified the T cell which killed and suppressed (i.e. $T_k$ and $T_s$). However, this tidy arrangement has been upset by observations (derived largely from the study of T cell clones) that some T4 positive cells can be cytotoxic and that suppressors can be T8 or T4 positive. A fact which has survived this recent reappraisal is that T4 cells always recognise antigen in association with **class II HLA** and T8 cells recognise antigen in association with **class I HLA**. It has been proposed that the T4 and T8 proteins are closely involved with the T cell receptor and interact directly with a non-polymorphic part of the respective HLA glycoproteins.

There is, nevertheless, functional heterogeneity within each of these two subsets. Helper cells are mostly T4 positive but some T4 cells can be cytotoxic against class II targets. T8 positivity identifies cells which are cytotoxic against class I targets as well as cells which act as effectors of suppression. $T_{dh}$ cells probably represent a differentiated form of T4 positive helper cell.

As much of the literature currently refers to $T_h$ and $T_k$ as clearly distinguishable subsets, I have retained this usage elsewhere in this book but the reader should be aware of the lack of complete equivalence with T4 and T8 positive cells.

## Dual recognition

Another feature which distinguishes T and B lymphocytes is that the former always recognise antigen in conjunction with HLA glycoproteins present on the surface of antigen-bearing cells: a phenomenon known as **dual recognition**. For the coincidental recognition of foreign antigen it is necessary that the HLA glycoprotein is of the same variety as that borne by 'self'. Much of the work on this phenomenon of HLA restriction has involved the use of virus-infected target cells. Virus-specific T cells are only able to kill virus-infected target cells if they share the same class I HLA glycoproteins with them (Fig. 3.2). Specific antibody, working in concert with complement or phagocytic cells, is usually effective in neutralising cell-free virus but is not able to eradicate viruses from within the cells in which the viruses are replicating. The main line of defence against virus-infected cells is the cytotoxic T cell and it is of considerable importance that this cell does not become activated by virus particles shed from cells but only develops lytic activity when it comes into direct contact with the infected cell.

A similar phenomenon is observed when T helper cells recognise antigen on the surface of antigen-presenting cells in association with class II HLA glycoproteins (Fig. 3.3) and, also, when T helper cells interact with B lymphocytes to cause them to proliferate into blast cells and divide to form antibody-secreting plasma cells. Thus, dual recognition of both antigen and self HLA glycoprotein guides the appropriate T cell to its target.

It may seem puzzling that antigen-bearing APC are not lysed by

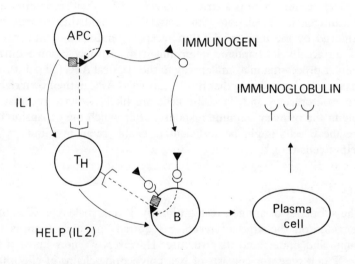

🁢 HLA class II

▶—○ immunogen containing carrier and hapten determinants

**Fig. 3.3** Dual recognition of antigen in association with class II HLA by the T4 positive helper cell. The initial step involves processing of the immunogen by the antigen-presenting cell (APC), which presents the carrier determinant in close proximity to the class II HLA glycoprotein. A T cell specific for this will, when stimulated by **interleukin 1** (IL-1) release, become activated to release its own growth factor, **interleukin 2** (IL-2). The B cell takes up the immunogen by its haptenic determinant and presents it to the T cell either by holding it on the surface or by processing it intracellularly so that it also is expressed in close proximity to class II HLA and recognised by the helper T cell. The release of IL-2 and other B cell growth factors then promotes the differentiation of the B cell into the antibody-secreting plasma cell.

killer T cells. However, this will be prevented by the specialised ability of the APC to take up, process and express antigen with class II rather than class I HLA and this may indicate the biological reason for this specialisation. Foreign (i.e. allogeneic) uninfected cells obtained from another genetically different member of the same species can be recognised in an allograft response — probably because they are seen as 'self + x' (see above and Chapter 14).

The combination of antigen presentation and interleukin 1 release by the APC causes the helper T cell to become activated and release its own growth factor, **interleukin 2** (IL-2) which stimulates other helper T cells, induces expression of the IL-2 receptor and also promotes the differentiation of B lymphocytes which have recognised the immunogen by its haptenic determinant.

Here again, there is a strict requirement for dual recognition of the antigen in association with class II HLA and this (a) may be achieved by the immunoglobulin receptor binding the antigen on its surface by its haptenic determinant or (b) may involve intracellular processing in a similar way to the classical APC (Fig. 3.3). It has recently been shown that B cells can act as APC in their own right but macrophages and dendritic cells are likely to have the major role in the primary immune response, after which the expansion of specific B cells might be sufficient to enable them to stimulate T helper cells directly.

### The T cell receptor

The subtleties of antigen recognition by T cells make considerable demands on the kind of receptor required and our attempts to define and understand its structure. However, we now know that the **T cell receptor** consists of two polypeptide chains of *c*. 50 000 MW ($\alpha$ chain) and *c*. 40 000 MW ($\beta$ chain) forming a heterodimer (Fig. 3.4). It is closely associated with the **CD3** glycoprotein which consists of three 20 000−25 000 MW subunits ($\gamma$, $\delta$ and $\varepsilon$). The $\alpha$ and $\beta$ chains of the heterodimer each contain a variable and a constant domain and are linked by a single disulphide bridge. $\alpha$ and $\beta$ chains show homology with both immunoglobulin and HLA glycoprotein molecules (Figs 3.4 and 4.3).

T cell receptors possess two different kinds of variable region and this creates considerable scope for the diversity of antigen recognition. There has been much debate concerning whether the dual recognition displayed by the T cell receptor is achieved by one receptor or by two separate receptors. Recent structural data deter-

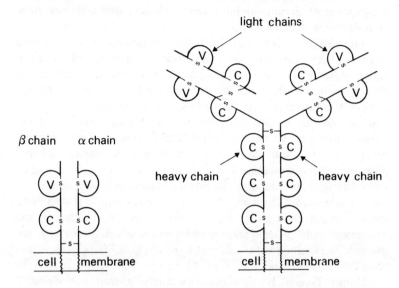

**Fig. 3.4** The structure of T and B cell receptors for antigen. Both the T cell receptor and the B cell receptor (consisting of monomeric IgM) have a similar domain structure to that found in the HLA glycoproteins (Fig. 4.3).

mined by DNA sequencing is in favour of a single receptor constructed of two similar but different polypeptide chains, each with their own kind of variability. The gene arrangements necessary to construct chains containing one out of many possible variable regions and one out of relatively few constant regions seem to be achieved in a similar way to that described for immunoglobulin molecules (see Chapter 5).

# B lymphocytes

The first specific recognition unit to be identified in the immune system was the immunoglobulin secreted by plasma cells. Their precursor cells — B lymphocytes — insert immunoglobulin molecules into their surface membrane, which can be detected by immunofluorescence. These molecules are the B cell receptor for antigen and contrast with the smaller T cell receptor (Fig. 3.4). The failure to detect immunoglobulin-like determinants on the surface of T cells by immunofluorescence is due to the fact that the anti-immunoglobulin reagents used are specific for the tail or Fc portion of immunoglobulin heavy chains, which do not form part of the T cell receptor.

The earliest cells of the B cell lineage can be detected in fetal liver and bone marrow. They lack surface immunoglobulin but can be identified by the presence of IgM heavy chains (i.e. μ chains) in their cytoplasm without detectable light chains (see p. 50). These are the **pre-B cells** which give rise to immature B cells expressing surface immunoglobulin which, initially, is of class IgM. Most resting B lymphocytes express both IgD and IgM but surface IgD is lost on antigenic stimulation and B memory cells lack this surface isotype. Further immunoglobulin class switches, i.e. to IgG, IgA or IgE, follow antigen stimulation. The mature **plasma cell** lacks all surface immunoglobulin. The nature of the stimulus which triggers immunoglobulin class switching is poorly understood although the immunoglobulin gene rearrangements by which different V genes are able to combine with different C region genes have been identified (see Figs 5.6 and 5.7).

Unlike T cells, B cell precursors emerging from haemopoietic tissue do not have to reside in a primary lymphoid organ such as the thymus to be able to differentiate into mature B lymphocytes. A consequence of this is that self-reactivity is still present within the B cell population although unbridled auto-immunity does not develop without the 'subversion' of relevant clones of T cells (see Chapter 10). When stimulated by appropriately presented antigen, B lymphocytes transform into activated blast cells which divide to form mature plasma cells secreting immunoglobulin into the extracellular fluids of the body. B cells also express class II HLA glycoproteins and receptors for Fc and C3. Various growth and differentiation factors have been described which govern the development of B cells, including interleukin 2 and gamma-interferon released by T helper cells. There is evidence for functional subdivision of the B cell population in man, e.g. some B cells preferentially recirculate and populate the follicles in lymph nodes and spleen whereas others are more static and localise to the marginal zones, and a number of surface markers have been identified.

Most lymphocytes are found within lymphoid tissues, e.g. lymph nodes, the white pulp of the spleen and mucosa-associated lymphoid tissue (MALT), i.e. lymphoid tissue present in the gut, the bronchial tree and mammary tissue. Both B and T lymphocytes actively recirculate and preferentially home to different parts of these tissues known, respectively, as T- and B-dependent areas.

# Lymph nodes

Lymphocytes gain entry to lymph nodes via two different routes: afferent lymphatics or the specialised high endothelial post-capillary venules present at the corticomedullary junction (Fig. 3.5). B lymphocytes are found predominantly in the outer cortex, which contains a number of denser aggregations of lymphocytes termed **follicles**. These enlarge during an active immune response to form **germinal centres**, which contain large numbers of proliferating B lymphoblasts surrounded by a mantle of resting small B lymphocytes. Antigens localise in germinal centres in the form of immune complexes and interact with follicular dendritic cells and the B cells that surround them. T lymphocytes, on the other hand, are diffusely present throughout the **paracortex** of the lymph node, where they interact with antigen on the surface of the interdigitating dendritic cells.

The co-operative event which takes place before B cells transform into antibody-secreting plasma cells may involve either direct cellular contact between the respective T and B cell populations at the junction of the T- and B-dependent areas or entry of T cells into the germinal centre itself. It is possible that most of the co-operative signals are transmitted by soluble factors diffusing across the interface between these two areas. Blast transformation of B cells is followed by the appearance of antibody-secreting plasma cells in the medulla of the lymph node and red pulp of the spleen with release of antibody into the efferent lymphatic and splenic veins, respectively.

# Spleen

The T- and B-dependent areas of the spleen are confined to the white pulp: the follicles and marginal zones are mostly occupied by B cells whereas the periarteriolar sheath almost entirely consists of T cells. The spleen has no lymphatic supply and splenic lymphocytes gain direct access to the circulation via the splenic vein.

# MALT

Unencapsulated mucosa-associated lymphoid tissue or MALT (which includes **tonsils, Peyer's patches, appendix** and **bronchial** and **mammary tissue**) contains many follicles but lymphocytes are also diffusely distributed in the **lamina propria** of the intestine

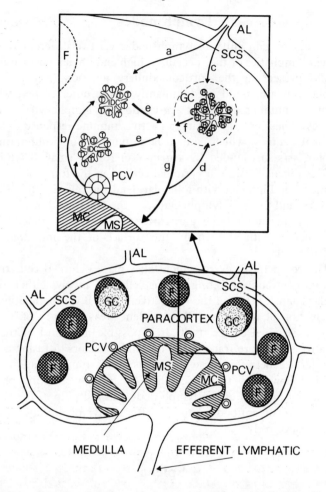

**Fig. 3.5 Lymph node structure and lymphocyte traffic.** The lower diagram shows
the overall structure of a lymph node with the cortical aggregations of B lymphocytes into **follicles** (F) and **germinal centres** (GC) and the subdivision of the
medulla into **medullary cords** (MC) and **medullary sinuses** (MS). T lymphocytes
are the predominant cell in the paracortex.

The upper diagram is an amplified inset of the cortex indicating the pathways by
which antigen gains access to the lymph node. This is either via **afferent lymphatics**
(AL) and the **subcapsular sinus** (SCS) (a and c) or via the **post-capillary venules**
(PCV) (b and d). Antigen in the form of immune complexes preferentially localises
to **follicular dendritic cells** (FDC) in the B cell-containing follicles or GC, whereas
antigen transported by dendritic cells in lymph (and possibly blood) is presented to
T helper cells in the paracortex which come into close contact with these **interdigitating dendritic cells** (IDC).

The process of T−B co-operation involves the approximation of these two kinds
of cell (e and f) and/or their soluble factors, culminating in the production of
B lymphoblasts which migrate (g) into the medullary cords and transform into
antibody-secreting plasma cells.

where only occasional follicles are present. Many of these lymphocytes have the characteristics of large granular lymphocytes (LGL)
and the gut is also well-endowed with its own variant of the mast
cell — mucosal mast cells.

## Lymphocyte circulation

There is a modest but steady transit of lymphocytes across the
venules of most tissues in the resting state. These cells migrate into
afferent lymphatics and gain access to lymph nodes via the marginal
sinus. The **post-capillary venules** (PCV) of lymphoid tissue have
specialised high endothelial cells which transfer large numbers of
lymphocytes directly from the blood into the lymph node when the
latter is actively stimulated (Fig. 3.5). The initial introduction of
antigen to the lymph node is probably via cells gaining entry
through the afferent lymph whereas the major ingress of lymphocytes during an active response is achieved directly via the PCV and
involves both non-specific and specific trapping of lymphocytes.

The normal circulatory patterns of T and B lymphocytes are
greatly modified during an active immune response and structures
on the surfaces of both lymphocytes and PCV determine the ability
of the former to migrate directly into lymphoid tissue. The period
of localised proliferation and differentiation of activated cells within
these specialised areas is associated with the renewal of their ability
to recirculate although they preferentially return to areas (mucosal
or non-mucosal) where they first encountered antigen. It is likely
that these 'educated' lymphocytes express surface receptors for
organ-specific endothelial determinants: B cells activated in gut-
associated lymphoid tissue are more likely to express receptors for
determinants on the surface of PCV present in that tissue and
preferentially return there. This is obviously of value in the defence
against infections acquired by a particular route and has particular
relevance to the newborn in view of the finding that mothers
challenged intestinally with antigen develop antibody-secreting cells
in mammary tissue and produce secretory IgA in their milk.

## Immunoregulation

The ability of the adaptive immune response to expand its store
of specifically reacting molecules and cells relevant to each successive antigenic experience is conserved by the presence of regulatory
factors which suppress the further expansion of specific immune

responses when they are no longer relevant. Much attention has
been paid to T cells which suppress specific responsiveness by an
inhibitory effect on the activity of T helper cells. Despite a great
deal of experimental work we still do not have a clear idea of the
identity of these cells or how they work (see p. 32).

All immune responses can be regarded as a balance between
help and suppression but it is not clear why most immune responses
start with help predominating and end with suppression to the fore.
If antigen comes into contact with T cells without having been
processed and presented by antigen-presenting cells, then, in this
free form, it is very likely to induce suppression. This may be
partly due to a tolerising effect on helper cells when they do not
receive the additional stimulation of interleukin 1 production by
APC. There is also evidence that suppressor cells may take longer
to become activated and may only become the predominant force in
the system when antigen has been largely eliminated.

## Differentiation pathways of the immune system

Figure 3.6 summarises the sequence by which stem cells differentiate into T and B subpopulations of lymphocytes which then
recirculate through the various lymphoid organs, lymph and peripheral blood. The lower part of the sequence requires the introduction of antigen presented by the various kinds of **antigen-
presenting cell** (APC). Further differentiation then takes place to
yield subpopulations of T and B cells able to release soluble factors,
i.e. interleukins, lymphokines and immunoglobulins, and which, in
the case of T killer cells, can have a direct cytotoxic effect on target
organisms or cells. Usually both cell-mediated and humoral immunity develop together but in some instances one of these arms of
the immune response may be activated disproportionately, e.g. in
some mycobacterial infections, a situation which has been called
'immune deviation'.

## Interleukins and lymphokines

T cells become activated following the release of **interleukin 1** (IL-
1) by the cells which present antigen to them. T4 cells then release
**interleukin 2** (IL-2), previously known as 'T cell growth factor',
which expands the pool of responding cells via an IL-2 receptor
expressed on activated T cells. Various factors have been described
which control the differentiation of B cells (e.g. B cell growth

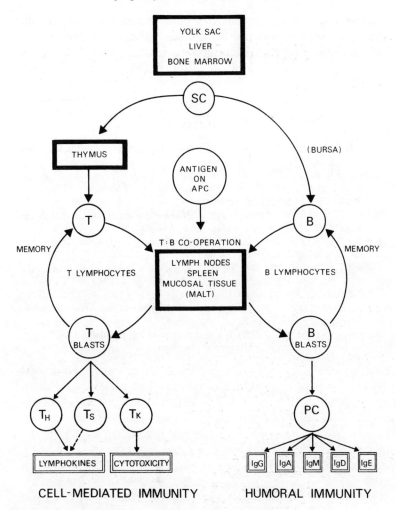

**Fig. 3.6** Differentiation pathways of the immune system.

factor — BCGF — and B cell differentiation factor — BCDF) but it is likely that IL-2 and gamma-interferon also have a role in B cell development. Growth factors are currently being defined for almost every kind of leucocyte and as their structure and function become completely understood it is likely that others will be categorised as interleukins. Candidates for IL-3 and IL-4 are currently under discussion.

**Lymphokine** is a generic term for biologically active soluble factors released by lymphocytes (and excludes immunoglobulin) but has been most often used to describe factors produced at sites of inflammation, e.g. macrophage activating factor (MAF), macrophage migration inhibition factor (MIF), chemotactic factors and cytotoxic factors.

## Further reading

Acuto O. & Reinherz E.L. (1985) The human T cell receptor. *New England Journal of Medicine*, **312**, 1110–11.

Benaceraff B. & Rock K.L. (1985) The significance of MHC restriction. In Medawar P. & Lehner T. eds. *The Gorer Symposium: the Major Histocompatibility System*. Blackwell Scientific Publications, Oxford.

Bernard A. *et al.* (1984) *Leucocyte Typing: Human Leucocyte Differentiation Antigens Detected by Monoclonal Antibodies*. Springer-Verlag, Berlin.

Butcher E.C. & Weissman I.L. (1984) Lymphoid tissues and organs. In Paul W.E. ed. *Fundamental Immunology*. Raven Press, New York.

Cannon J.G. & Dinarello C.A. (1987) The nature of interleukins. In Thompson R.A. ed. *Recent Advances in Clinical Immunology*, 4. Churchill Livingstone, Edinburgh.

Feldmann M. (1985) Lymphokines and interleukins emerge from the primeval soup. *Nature*, **313**, 351–3.

Fossum S. & Ford W.L. (1985) The organization of cell populations within lymph nodes: their origin, life history and functional relationships. *Histopathology*, **9**, 469–99.

# Chapter 4
## The HLA system and its proteins

Considerable interest in the biochemical uniqueness of the individual followed the introduction of organ transplantation in the 1960s. Although blood group antigen systems were already well-defined it soon became clear that the individual tissue type was of paramount importance in determining the rate and severity of graft rejection. The exchange of tissue between genetically identical members of the same species, i.e. **syngeneic** or **isologous** transfers, are tolerated indefinitely whereas the exchange of tissue between genetically different members of the same species, i.e. **allogeneic** or **homologous** transfers, and between members of different species, i.e. **xenogeneic** or **heterologous** transfers, are both followed by the development of graft-reactive T cells and antibody culminating in rejection of the foreign tissue. This terminology is summarised in Fig. 4.1. The commonest transfers performed in man are those of tissues or organs obtained from living or cadaveric human donors, i.e. **allografts** (previously called homografts), for which the rejection process has to be subdued by the use of immunosuppressive drugs. The proteins on the surface of cells which are recognised as 'foreign'

| RELATIONSHIP | NOUNS | ADJECTIVES | |
|---|---|---|---|
| 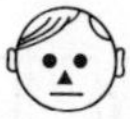 | Autograft | Syngeneic | Autologous |
| 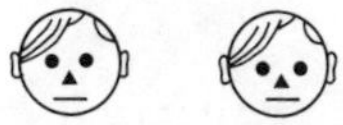 | Isograft | Syngeneic | Isologous |
| 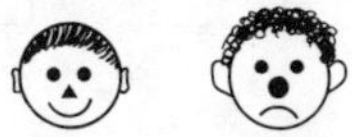 | Allograft | Allogeneic | Homologous |
| 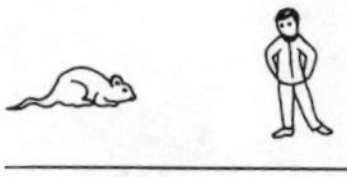 | Xenograft | Xenogeneic | Heterologous |

**Fig. 4.1** Terms used to describe immunological relationships.

43

and the genes that code for their many varieties constitute the major histocompatibility system (MHS) or complex (MHC).

## The mouse H2 system

The major histocompatibility system in mice (known as H2) was defined by exchanging skin grafts between members of different inbred strains and observing how the incidence and severity of rejection related to the genetic background of these animals. Two major loci were identified on chromosome 17 and designated K and D (Fig. 4.2). Later, it became clear that animals who were identical at the K and D loci were often able to express immunological difference which were detected in other ways.

Firstly, if lymphocytes from one strain were incubated in a **mixed lymphocyte culture** (MLC) with the lymphocytes of another strain showing identity at K and D, then these lymphocytes would often stimulate each other in this *in vitro* assay. The differences that the lymphocytes were detecting were shown to be due to the presence of other proteins under the control of genes in the I region located within the left-hand half of the mouse MHC, i.e. extending from the K locus to the locus for the fourth complement component (Fig. 4.2). These are often referred to as **Ia genes** (immune associated). Secondly, animals which only differ in the I region may also show striking differences in their ability to produce antibody to well-defined synthetic antigens, e.g. random co-polymers of amino

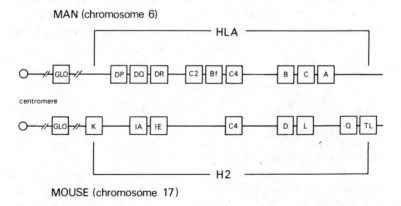

**Fig. 4.2** Genetic maps of the major histocompatibility complex (MHC) in man and the mouse. See text for definition of the various loci. GLO is the glyoxalase locus — a useful non-MHC marker.

acids such as tyrosine−glutamic acid−arginine−lysine (TGAL). These differences in responsiveness were also shown to segregate with genes within the I region known as immune response or **Ir genes.**

## The human HLA system

The unravelling of the human MHC has largely been achieved by documenting protein variations on the surfaces of peripheral blood leucocytes; hence the term Human Leucocyte Antigen or HLA system. Multiple pregnancies or blood transfusions often induce antibodies to these HLA proteins and sera from such individuals have been used to type for these proteins. This is why these HLA proteins are also referred to as 'antigens'. The first loci to be described were **HLA-A** and **HLA-B** (Fig. 4.2) followed by a third minor locus designated **HLA-C**. However, when lymphocytes were obtained from two individuals identical at these major histocompatibility loci it was found that they were still able to stimulate each other in a mixed lymphocyte culture. This led to the mapping of a further locus, **HLA-D**, which has since been shown to code for glycoproteins equivalent to the Ia polymorphisms of the mouse.

The human MHC also contains genes for several complement components, i.e. C4, C2 and factor B (Bf), and there is close homology between the human and murine MHC gene complexes (Fig. 4.2) except that most of the major loci (HLA-A and HLA-B) are to the right of the complex in man whereas one of the major loci in the mouse (K) is to the left of the I region. It is possible that this disparity arose by a chromosomal cross-over during evolution for in all other respects these two arrangements are remarkably similar.

## Class I glycoproteins

These are the major histocompatibility antigens which are present on all nucleated cells, i.e. H2-K and H2-D in the mouse and HLA-A, HLA-B and HLA-C in man. Their overall structure shows considerable similarity with the other important surface proteins involved in immune recognition, i.e. class II glycoproteins, T cell receptors, B cell receptors and secreted immunoglobulins (see Figs 4.3, 3.4 and 5.5). Class I glycoproteins consist of a large $\alpha$ polypeptide chain and a smaller polypeptide known as $\beta2$ microglobulin ($\beta2M$). The former contains three peptide loops designated $\alpha1$, $\alpha2$ and $\alpha3$ with the lowermost part of the $\alpha$ chain extending through

CLASS I HLA        CLASS II HLA

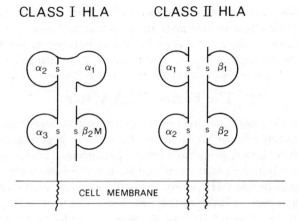

Fig. 4.3 Structure of class I and class II HLA glycoproteins.

the cell membrane into the cytoplasm. The single loop or domain of β2 microglobulin is non-covalently linked to the α chain on the surface of the cell. The α1 and α2 domains contain the variable part of the class I glycoprotein, which confers a major part of the uniqueness of the individual on every nucleated cell. The physiological function of these molecules is to enable T lymphocytes of the killer subset ($T_k$) to interact successfully with self cells which bear foreign antigens upon their surface in association with class I glycoproteins, i.e. the phenomenon of **dual recognition** (see p. 32). This particularly applies to virus-infected cells where it would be inappropriate, and often impossible, for killer T cells to inactivate free virus particles but where the crucial requirement is for virus-infected cells — an important source of new virus particles — to be eliminated as effectively as possible. This form of immune guidance means that T killer cells are only triggered when they see both antigen and class I glycoprotein in close association (see Fig. 3.2). The same principle underlies reactivity towards allogeneic cells in which specific T cells see this kind of foreignness as 'self + x' — T cells that react with self alone having been eliminated as part of the thymic censoring process (see p. 29).

## Class II glycoproteins

The expression of these molecules is confined to cells directly involved in immune responses, i.e. macrophages, other antigen-presenting cells, e.g. dendritic cells and Langerhans cells, T helper cells and B cells (Table 2.3 and Fig. 3.3). Class II molecules show some similarity in overall structure with their class I counterparts except that the α and β chains are of similar size (33 000 and 28 000 MW respectively); each contains two polypeptide domains and traverses the cell membrane and together they form a heterodimer (Fig. 4.3). Most of the structural variation between individuals is contained within the β chain but some class II proteins also possess variation in their α chain.

The physiological role of class II HLA glycoproteins is to provide appropriate guidance for T helper cells in their interaction with antigen-presenting cells, on the one hand, and B lymphocytes, on the other, with both of which successful interaction takes place during an immune response. It would clearly be inappropriate for T helper cells to be triggered and release interleukin 2 by contact with other antigen-bearing cells although it has recently been realised that other tissue cells, e.g. thyrocytes and liver cells, can express class II proteins during acute inflammation, probably due to the local release of interferon. This may have a physiological role in increasing the scope for antigen presentation to incoming T helper cells.

The production of monoclonal antibodies specific for HLA proteins and the analysis of the DNA sequences that code for them has shown that the human equivalent to the I region in the mouse is rather more complex than was at first thought. HLA-D typing is now usually achieved by the use of serological reagents and peripheral blood B cells which bear adequate quantities of class II glycoproteins. The series of antigens detected by this means is referred to as **DR** (D-related). Many of these coincide with the D specificities determined by MHC typing and both series are now well into double figures in terms of the number of possible alternatives.

Some antisera detect determinants shared by more than one DR type and are termed supertypic specificities. This has led to the definition of another class II locus designated **DQ** (previously DC) in close proximity to DR (Fig. 4.4). A further closely linked locus — **DP** — has been defined on the basis of secondary stimulation in mixed lymphocyte culture (known as primed lymphocyte typing) although the number of possible alternatives at these other two loci is still in single figures. The DR region has one α and three β genes, and both DQ and DP regions each contain two α and two β genes. However, DNA sequencing indicates that there are at least six genes for class II α chain proteins and at least seven genes for class II β chain proteins: so it is likely that a further locus exists (currently designated DX). An individual heterozygous for class II

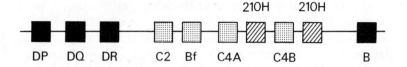

**Fig. 4.4** Expanded version of part of the HLA complex.

genes will be able to form a number of $\alpha-\beta$ heterodimers by virtue of the different combinations which may be possible between the products of different gene loci that he or she possesses. This helps to explain the considerable polymorphism of these class II proteins although it appears that some haplotypes (see p. 187) express a smaller number of class II genes than others.

The sequence of the other genes which lie between HLA-DR and HLA-B is shown in Fig. 4.4. The three complement components, C2, C4 and factor B, are each involved in the generation of enzymes capable of activating the bulk reaction of the complement pathway, i.e. C3 conversion. The genes for C4 have become reduplicated to form two loci C4A and C4B and these lie beside duplicated loci for an enzyme involved in the 21-hydroxylation of steroids (21OH). This enzyme is deficient in congenital adrenal hyperplasia — a condition which shows a strong association with a particular HLA haplotype in which both C4 and 21-hydroxylase are deficient. The link between the HLA system and disease is reviewed in Chapter 15.

The complement protein loci are sometimes referred to as class III genes and their products also show polymorphism. This is most marked at the C4A and C4B loci and their molecular variations are associated with variation in the functional performance of these proteins. The most extreme form of this is the occurrence of null genes which fail to give rise to a recognisable complement protein. Other class I-like genes have been identified to the right of HLA-A (resembling Q and TL loci in the mouse) (see Fig. 4.2). Their proteins have been identified on the surface of human lymphocytes and are regarded as differentiation antigens although their actual function is unknown.

## Further reading

Bach F.H. (1985) The HLA class II genes and products: the HLA-D region. *Immunology Today*, **6**, 89–94.
Bodmer W.F. (1984) The HLA system. In Albert E.D. *et al*. eds. *Histocompatibility Testing 1984*. Springer-Verlag, Berlin.

# Chapter 5
# Immunoglobulins

All vertebrates possess immunoglobulin-like molecules. They are synthesised and secreted by end cells of the B cell lineage, i.e. plasma cells. These serum proteins were first discovered a century ago by Paul Ehrlich and his colleagues by virtue of their ability to confer protection, i.e. immunity, against a number of important bacterial infections. They are largely confined to the broad and heterogeneous band of γ-globulins observed on electrophoresis (Fig. 5.1) and show considerable diversity of structure and function.

## Structure

The typical immunoglobulin molecule is asymmetrically composed of four polypeptide chains linked by disulphide bridges (Fig. 5.2). The larger chains are designated **heavy** and the smaller **light** and it is the combined N-terminal ends of these two chains (on the left in Fig. 5.2) which create the two antigen-binding sites of the

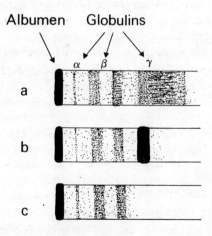

**Fig. 5.1** Protein electrophoresis of (a) normal serum, (b) serum showing a compact band of monoclonal immunoglobulin (from a case of myeloma) and (c) serum from a patient with hypogammaglobulinaemia.

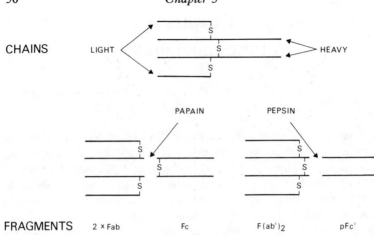

CHAINS

FRAGMENTS     2 × Fab              Fc              F(ab')₂          pFc'

**Fig. 5.2** Immunoglobulin chains and the fragments formed by proteolytic digestion.

molecule. The right-hand or C-terminal portion of the molecule mediates various effector functions which are triggered following combination of the immunoglobulin molecule with its specific antigen. Several immunoglobulin fragments can be prepared using proteolytic enzymes and these have been of value in unravelling the functional activities of different parts of these molecules. **Fab** was designated thus because it was the fragment that retained the ability to recognise antigen — a classical feature of antibody (ab) molecules — following digestion with papain. The other fragment could be readily crystallised and was thus termed **Fc**. Pepsin digestion cleaves the molecule to the right-hand side of the 'hinge' region and this generates an Fab dimer designated F (ab')₂, leaving a rather smaller Fc fragment designated pFc'. Even more of the Fc portion is retained within the Fab fragment derived by plasmin treatment and this is designated Fabc.

**Variable and constant domains**

Figure 5.3 illustrates the immunoglobulin molecule in a Y configuration and emphasises the flexible hinge region which permits considerable movement of the Fab arms. Both light and heavy polypeptide chains consist of a series of similar subunits or **domains**. Each domain consists of a stretch of *c.* 110 amino acids held

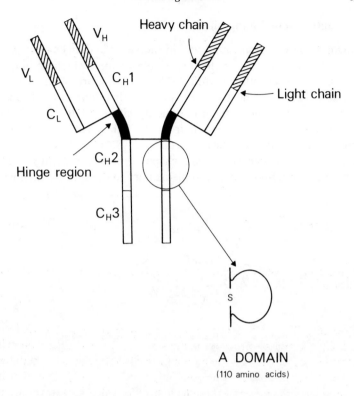

**A DOMAIN**
(110 amino acids)

**Fig. 5.3** The domain structure of immunoglobulin molecules. See text.

in a single loop by an intrachain disulphide bridge. Although there is considerable overall similarity between the various light and heavy chain domains, the N-terminal domain shows a marked degree of variation of many of its amino acid residues and is termed **variable** in contrast to the other domains which vary comparatively little from each other and are termed **constant**. Light chains contain one variable and one constant domain ($V_L$ and $C_L$) whereas heavy chains contain one variable region ($V_H$) and three or four constant region domains ($C_H1$, $C_H2$, $C_H3$ and $C_H4$) depending on the class of immunoglobulin. The domain structure of immunoglobulins is very similar to the pattern of polypeptide looping found in T cell receptors (Fig. 3.4) as well as that seen in both kinds of HLA glycoprotein (Fig. 4.3). This suggests that they have all developed as specialisations of an ancestral recognition molecule present upon the surface of most kinds of cell.

## The antigen-combining site

Much of the variation found within the variable domains is located within three 'hot spots' or **hypervariable regions** which lie in close proximity to each other within the folded structure of the variable domain. Thus, the most variable parts of this domain are brought together to form the **antigen-combining site** or cleft consisting of the three hypervariable regions from the light chain and a further three from the adjacent heavy chain (Fig. 5.4a).

The specific chemistry and shape of this combining site is termed the **paratope** and is complementary to the specific chemistry

$V_L$  $V_L$  $V_L$

CLEFT

$V_H$  $V_H$  $V_H$

(a) Formation of the antigen combining cleft or paratope from the six constituent hypervariable regions

EPITOPE

PARATOPE

(b) Interaction between an antigen epitope and the antibody cleft (in transverse section)

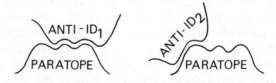

ANTI - $ID_1$

PARATOPE

ANTI-$ID_2$

PARATOPE

(c) Interaction between anti-idiotype antibodies of two different specificities (anti-$id_1$ and anti-$id_2$) and the idiotypic region of the antibody molecule (in transverse section)

**Fig. 5.4** Spatial configuration of the antigen-combining site or cleft and its interaction with epitopes or other idiotypes.

and shape of the **epitope** or antigenic determinant (Fig. 5.4b and Chapter 2). The term paratope is confined to that part of the molecule which specifically interacts with the epitope, whereas the entire area of surface conformation which is unique to a particular molecule is known as the **idiotype**. These unique shapes and surfaces can themselves be recognised by other antibodies which are then referred to as having **anti-idiotype** specificity (Fig. 5.4c). If they interact sufficiently with the antigen-combining site, they may block the combination of antigen epitope with it (e.g. anti-id$_1$) or, if they react with a more peripheral part, they may not inhibit epitope combination (e.g. anti-id$_2$).

### Affinity and avidity

The strength of binding or association of a single epitope for a single paratope in a homogeneous system is termed **affinity**. The more usual situation whereby an antigen bearing several epitopes combines with a variety of specific antibody molecules, each with their own paratopes, is a very heterogeneous system and the term **avidity** is used to indicate the average strength of this association. The former is as easy to measure as the strength of binding of a hormone for its receptor: the latter is a much more complicated affair.

# Classes and subclasses

There are five classes of immunoglobulin in man: IgG, IgA, IgM, IgD and IgE (Table 5.1 and Fig. 5.5). These show important structural and functional differences and, in the case of IgG and IgA, subdivide further into subclasses. Each of these structural variants is present in all normal individuals. They can be identified and quantified by specific antisera raised in another species and are referred to as **isotypes**. Other, single amino acid, variations occur as heritable polymorphisms and are known as **allotypes**. These have been identified within IgG (the Gm system), IgA (the Am system) and on K chains (the Km system) and are coded for by genes on chromosomes 14, 11 and 2, respectively.

Each class (or subclass) of immunoglobulin consists of four-chain units as depicted in Figs 5.3 and 5.5. In IgG, IgD and IgE, these are monomeric whereas IgA often occurs as a dimer and IgM almost always as a pentamer. The heavy chains of each class are

**Table 5.1** Physical and biological characteristics of immunoglobulins.

| | IgG | IgA | IgM | IgD | IgE |
|---|---|---|---|---|---|
| **Physical properties** | | | | | |
| Molecular weight | 150 000 | 160 000 (monomer) | 900 000 | 180 000 | 190 000 |
| Number of four-chain units | 1 | 1 or 2 | 5 | 1 | 1 |
| Heavy chains | γ | α | μ | δ | ε |
| Light chains | κ or λ | κ or λ | κ or λ | κ or λ | κ or λ |
| Other peptide chains | – | J[a] ± S[b] | J[a] | – | – |
| Subclasses | γ1 γ2 γ3 γ4 | α1 α2 | – | – | – |
| Serum concentration (g l$^{-1}$) | c. 10 (65% 25% 6% 4%) | c. 2 (85% 15%) | c. 1 | c. 0·03 | c. 0·0002 (i.e. 200 ng ml$^{-1}$) |
| **Biological activities** | | | | | |
| Complement fixation: | | | | | |
| Classical pathway | γ1 γ2 γ3 | – | ++ | – | – |
| Alternative pathway | +[c] | + | – | – | – |
| Phagocyte binding | γ1 γ3 | +[d] | – | – | +[d] |
| Mast cell binding | – | – | – | – | ++ |
| Placental transfer | γ1 γ2 γ3 γ4 | – | – | – | – |

[a]J = J chain. [b]S = secretory piece. [c]See text. [d]See Table 7.4.

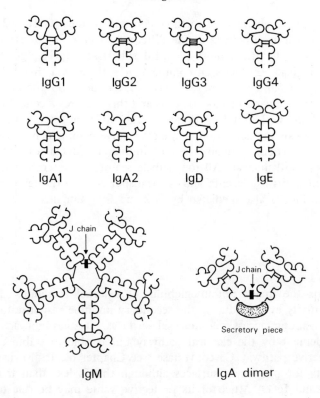

IgG1   IgG2   IgG3   IgG4

IgA1   IgA2   IgD   IgE

J chain

Secretory piece

IgM        IgA dimer

**Fig. 5.5** Structure of immunoglobulin isotypes.

given the equivalent Greek letter, e.g. γ for IgG (see Table 5.1). The light chains can be of two types, kappa (κ) or lambda (λ) and the two light chains of a single immunoglobulin molecule are of the same type, i.e. *either* κ *or* λ. Both polymeric forms (IgA and IgM) contain an additional peptide known as **J chain** (15 000 MW) which plays a part in holding the monomeric subunits together. Dimeric IgA, present in secretions, contains a further component known as **secretory piece** (70 000 MW) which is derived from cells of the secretory epithelium through which IgA is transported.

## IgG

This is the most plentiful immunoglobulin in internal body fluids and is produced particularly during the secondary immune response. The γ chains contain three constant regions (Cγ1, Cγ2 and Cγ3) which are involved in the different effector functions of the molecule. The three most plentiful subclasses (IgG1, IgG2 and IgG3) activate the classical complement pathway via the Cγ2 domain (see Chapter 6). Only subclasses IgG1 and IgG3 interact with the Fc receptor on phagocytic cells and this requires a contribution from both Cγ2 and Cγ3 domains. IgG in aggregated form can enhance existing activation of the alternative complement pathway but the particular involvement of individual subclasses and domains is still unclear. All four subclasses of IgG interact with Fc receptors in the placenta and are transported into the fetal circulation. This is also mediated by Cγ2 and Cγ3 domains.

## IgA

This is the major immunoglobulin of external secretions. It is particularly evident during the secondary immune response to antigen gaining access via mucosal surfaces. It does not activate complement by the classical pathway but is able to stabilise the alternative pathway C3 convertase (see Chapter 6). It also has an affinity for phagocyte surfaces although this is less than that of IgG1 and IgG3. Much of its protective value may be due to its direct combination with and neutralisation of pathogenic microorganisms in the gut and respiratory tract without necessarily involving any other effector systems.

IgA dimers and their associated **J chains** are produced by submucosal plasma cells. They gain access to the lumen of the gut and other mucosal sites by complexing with a receptor for polymeric immunoglobulin present on the surface of enterocytes and hepatocytes. This receptor has a high affinity for J chain and, after combination with it, dimeric IgA is transported across the cell by endocytosis and then released with the outer portion of the poly-Ig receptor still attached. This component which forms an important part of secretory IgA is designated **secretory piece**.

Dimeric, J chain-containing, IgA also gains access to the portal circulation and is transported into bile via the poly-Ig receptor present on hepatocytes. As most circulating IgA in man (in contrast to mice and rats) is present in monomeric form it is unlikely that this is an important route for the transport of secretory IgA into the gut under normal conditions.

## IgM

This is the key immunoglobulin of the primary response and is a large pentameric molecule containing ten antigen-combining sites, the five monomeric units being linked together with a single J chain molecule. Its heavy (μ) chains have four constant domains (Fig. 5.5). IgM is an efficient activator of the classical complement pathway. The level of specific antibody belonging to this class fades with progressive exposure to specific antigen in favour of other isotypes, e.g. IgG and IgA. T cells are thought to have a role in governing the mechanism of isotype switching, and the nature of the immuno-globulin gene arrangements which mediate this event are described below. J chain-containing IgM also has an affinity for the poly-Ig receptor and when there is a relative dearth of IgA, as in IgA deficiency, then IgM can appear in secretions linked to secretory piece.

## IgD

This is normally present in minute concentrations in blood and other body fluids but is readily detected on the surface of many early B cells in conjunction with IgM. It is not thought to mediate any of the usual effector functions attributed to immunoglobulin but may have a role as antigen receptor on early B cells.

## IgE

This monomeric immunoglobulin has four constant domains (like IgM) and, although it is the least plentiful of all immunoglobulins, its presence can be dramatically felt by its ability to bind to Fc receptors on the surface of mast cells and basophils and, when complexed with specific antigen, to trigger the release of inflam-matory mediators (see Chapter 8). Its physiological role may be to function with mast cells as a 'gatekeeper' regulating the exit of cells and plasma into extravascular sites. Its ability to bind to the surface of phagocytic cells, e.g. macrophages, may also be important in immunity to parasites.

## Triggering of effector systems

In some situations antibodies can act alone, e.g. neutralisation of bacterial toxins and viruses and inhibition of flagellar motility.

However, their effect is most striking when they are able to trigger and recruit the assistance of other effector molecules and cells, e.g. complement and phagocytes (Table 1.2). Clearly, it would be inappropriate for this event to be mediated by uncomplexed immunoglobulin and strict requirements have to be fulfilled before the appropriate signal is generated. For activation of the classical complement pathway by IgG, two adjacent IgG molecules have to be stabilised within an immune complex or IgG aggregate and at an appropriate distance from each other such that a minimum of two of the six heads of the first complement protein (Clq) can interact with the C$\gamma$2 domain which then causes a steric rearrangement of the C1 complex with activation of C1r and C1s (see Chapter 6). Each of the other domains in the IgG molecule is stabilised by a hydrophobic interaction with its homologous partner whereas the C$\gamma$2 domains are partly masked by carbohydrate and protrude outward, facilitating their interaction with Clq.

Each of the other effector functions, e.g. phagocyte activation and mast cell degranulation, is also triggered by the approximation and stabilisation of Fc domains within complexed antibody. The requirement for cross-linking of surface IgE on the mast cell has been shown by the demonstration that mast cell degranulation can be produced by intact divalent anti-IgE but not with monovalent Fab fragments of this reagent.

## Immunoglobulin genes

It was a source of puzzlement for many years how, if each protein (or polypeptide chain) is under the control of a single gene, immunoglobulin molecules with identical constant regions but different variable regions could be synthesised. The discovery of intervening sequences (IVS) or **introns** as well as coding sequences or **exons** within chromosomal DNA and the realisation that rearrangements of these sequences were possible have helped to clarify this problem.

It was always difficult to comprehend how up to $10^8$ different antibody specificities could be coded by genes inherited in the germ-line but it is now clear that many of the rearrangements of DNA and RNA that take place during B cell differentiation make a significant contribution to the total diversity of the antibody molecules which are produced. Figure 5.6 illustrates the way in which rearrangements are made in the germ-line DNA coding for lambda light chain proteins such that one (e.g. $V_1$) of a number of variable

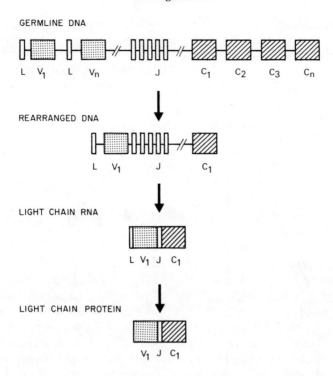

**Fig. 5.6** Organisation and rearrangement of genes coding for lambda light chains.

region genes is rearranged adjacent to a series of joining (J) genes prior to RNA splicing to a single constant region gene (e.g. $C_1$). The DNA for kappa chains contains only one constant region gene although the process of $V-J-C$ joining is otherwise identical.

Further diversity is possible with the rearrangements that take place in the DNA coding for heavy chains (Fig. 5.7). In addition to a considerable number of variable region genes there is also a group of diversity (D) genes which code for the third hypervariable region of the heavy chain. The first step in DNA rearrangement is for a single variable region gene ($V_1$) to be linked through one of several diversity genes to the J gene cluster prior to linkage to the constant region gene for IgM or IgD ($C\mu$ or $C\delta$) by RNA splicing.

The eight other constant region genes occur in two groups of four. They are likely to have arisen by tandem gene duplication and the primordial gene cluster probably took the form: $C\mu/C\delta$ followed by $C\gamma$, $C\epsilon$ and $C\alpha$. The mechanism whereby these other constant

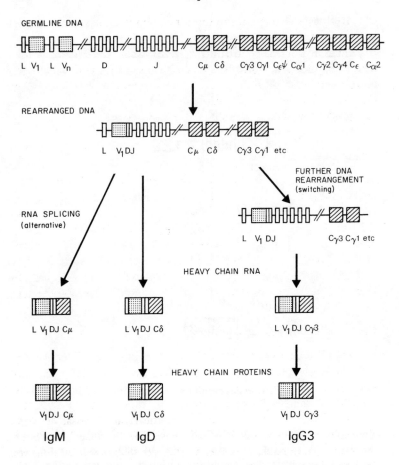

**Fig. 5.7** Organisation and rearrangement of genes coding for heavy chains.

region genes, i.e. Cγ3 to Cα2, can be linked to the same variable region genes as Cμ or Cδ is thought to be under the control of 'switch' sequences of DNA. This enables longer loops of DNA to be removed and constant region genes for IgG, IgE and IgA to be located in close proximity to variable region genes (Fig. 5.7).

It is not yet clear what causes one switch sequence to have preference over another and how T lymphocytes are involved in the process of isotype switching. During the process of B lymphocyte differentiation the heavy chain genes are rearranged first, followed by the light chain genes (kappa before lambda), with subsequent exclusion of either κ or λ genes from the expressed product of the cell. Exclusion also applies to immunoglobulin allotypes as each cell only expresses one allele.

Thus, at least three genes code for a **light chain** and four for a **heavy chain** with a total of **seven genes** coding for a complete **immunoglobulin protein**. Other classes of antibody which contain identical variable regions are produced by rearranging the sets of light and heavy chain genes as described above.

## Origin of diversity

Several factors contribute to the enormous range of antibody diversity present in higher vertebrates. Firstly, multiple V region genes are present in the **germ-line**. The ability to use either of two **light chain gene sets** creates further diversity. **Somatic mutation** creates other possibilities during the many cell divisions that take place in the B cell lineage. Lastly, **recombination**, particularly between V and J genes for light chains and V, D and J genes for heavy chains, offers further scope for variation in the final product.

## Clonal selection vs. instruction

Before the above mechanisms for creating antibody diversity were identified, it had been proposed that pluripotential cells were 'instructed' to synthesise a particular kind of antibody molecule following contact with specific antigen in order to produce a matching specificity of antibody. However, the rival proposal of **clonal selection** is now regarded as the basis of the adaptive immune response. In essence, this means that those lymphocytes bearing receptors that fit the epitope best are preferentially stimulated to divide and produce more cells of the same specificity. It is extremely unusual for only one kind of receptor, i.e. specificity, to be stimulated with the result that a hierarchy of cells is triggered, giving rise to a **polyclonal** response consisting of antibody molecules with a range of affinities for the epitopes concerned. The antibodies produced in a secondary response are likely to be of higher affinity in view of preferential expansion of those clones which best fit the antigen.

**Monoclonal** or **oligoclonal** responses are usually seen in abnormal situations, e.g. myelomatosis, during recovery following a bone marrow graft or when antibody-producing cells are fused experimentally with plasmacytoma cells *in vitro* to form a monoclonal hybridoma.

## Antigen—antibody combination

Antigens and antibodies do not combine in fixed proportions, i.e. their union is not stoichiometric. This is illustrated in a standard **quantitative precipitation test** (Fig. 5.8) in which increasing concentrations of antigen are added to a series of tubes containing a constant concentration of antibody. A maximum amount of precipitate is formed at an optimum point but antigen—antibody complexes form at other numerical proportions of antigen and antibody. These complexes vary in their composition: complexes formed near the point of optimal proportions or **equivalence** are largest and tend to form a lattice whereas those formed in antibody excess or antigen excess are smaller and precipitate less readily. This method

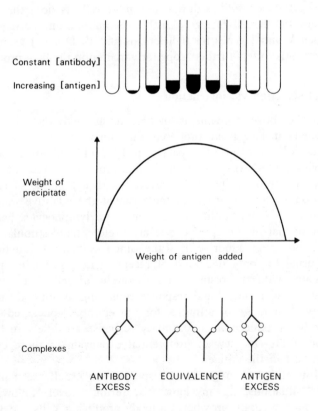

**Fig. 5.8** The quantitative precipitin test showing the variation in amount of precipitate formed and the size of complexes at different antigen—antibody ratios.

can be used to determine the amount of antibody present in an antiserum as well as the valency of the antigen.

## Laboratory methods

These principles underlie many different kinds of **immunodiffusion** technique in which antigens and antibodies diffuse toward each other through a transparent support medium, e.g. agar, to form lines of precipitation in the equivalence zone (Fig. 5.9). These methods are used to detect and characterize solutions or extracts of antigens or antibodies (e.g. **double diffusion**), to measure the concentration of a particular protein antigen (e.g. **radial immuno-diffusion**), to detect qualitative differences in proteins present in serum or other fluids (e.g. **immuno-electrophoresis** — and see Fig. 13.2) and to quantify proteins differentially (**two-dimensional immuno-electrophoresis**).

The coupling of antigens to the surface of red cells or other particles provides greater sensitivity for the detection of specific

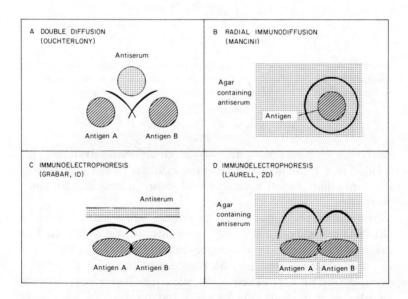

**Fig. 5.9** Immunodiffusion techniques for characterising specific antigens or antibodies.

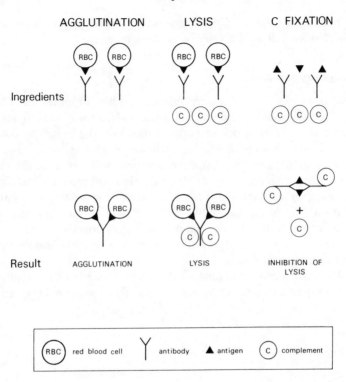

**Fig. 5.10** Agglutination, lysis and complement fixation techniques for detecting specific antibodies. Results are often reported as a titre, i.e. the weakest dilution of serum which gives a positive result.

antibodies by **agglutination, lysis** or **complement fixation** (Fig. 5.10). These techniques still form the mainstay of blood grouping, cross-matching and the detection of many microbial and auto-antibodies.

**Immunofluorescence**, and techniques using enzyme-labelled (**ELISA**) and radio-labelled (**RIA**) reagents are also widely used to determine the specificity of antigen-antibody reactions (Fig. 5.11) and to examine tissues for the presence of immunological components (see p. 121). Their applications are legion but, as with all laboratory methods, the accuracy and precision of the results obtained depend on the regular use of internal and external standards and the rigorous application of quality control protocols.

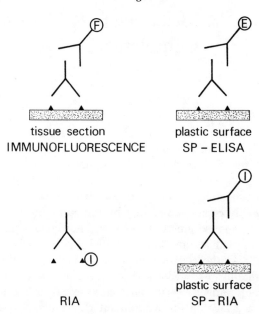

**Fig. 5.11** Other indicator systems for detecting specific antibody. Immunofluorescent techniques involve the reaction of antibody with sections of antigen-containing tissue. After suitable washing, the antibody can be detected using a fluorescein-labelled second antibody (i.e. antiglobulin) and UV microscopy. The solid-phase enzyme-linked immunosorbent assay (SP-ELISA) utilises antigen-coated plastic tubes or wells. Antibody binding is detected using an enzyme-conjugated antiglobulin and the colour generated on addition of substrate is read visually or with a spectrophotometer. Radio-immunoassay (RIA) is more often used to determine amounts of antigen (e.g. hormone) and is a measure of how much of a standard amount of radio-labelled antigen is displaced from antibody binding in the presence of the unknown material. Solid-phase RIA is exactly comparable to SP-ELISA except that a radio-labelled antiglobulin is used and the amount of antibody bound is determined by $\gamma$ counting.

# Further reading

French M.A.H. ed. (1986) *Immunoglobulins in Health and Disease.* MTP Press, Lancaster.

Honjo T. (1983) Immunoglobulin genes. *Annual Review of Immunology,* **1**, 499–528.

Klein J. (1982) Immunoglobulins and B cell receptors. In *Immunology: the Science of Self: Non-self Discrimination.* Wiley, Chichester.

Rose N.R., Friedman H. & Fahey J.L. eds (1986) *Manual of Clinical Laboratory Immunology,* 3rd edn. American Society for Microbiology, Washington.

Underdown B.J. & Schiff J.M. (1986) Immunoglobulin A: strategic defense initiative at the mucosal surface. *Annual Review of Immunology,* **4**, 384–417.

# Chapter 6
# Complement

The presence of serum factors which could augment the effects of antigen–antibody combination was first detected by Jules Bordet almost 100 years ago. He showed that serum containing a red cell antibody would cause lysis of red cells when it was fresh but only agglutination when aged. The material which *complemented* the effect of antibody could be restored by the addition of fresh non-antibody-containing serum and is now known to consist of a number of different serum proteins which operate as an enzyme cascade similar to the coagulation system. Table 6.1 summarises the original findings of Bordet and indicates that when an extraneous source of antigen–antibody complexes is introduced less complement is available for fixation on the antibody-coated red cells and less lysis is observed. This is the basis of the traditional **complement fixation test** in which test serum is incubated with the relevant antigen and a standard dose of complement, followed by a second stage in which the amount of complement consumed is determined by the degree of red cell lysis (see Fig. 5.10).

Until recently, most attention was focused upon the lytic ability of the complement system but this is now known to be only one of several important biological effects of complement activation. Most of these involve the activation or fixation of the third complement component (C3) and this can be achieved in two different ways: by **activation** of the **classical pathway** or by **stabilisation** of the **alternative pathway** (Fig. 6.1). If these initial steps take place on a cell or basement membrane then complement activation will proceed

**Table 6.1** Incubation of red cells with combinations of antibody, complement (C) and other antigen–antibody (Ag–Ab) complexes.

| RBC | RBC antibody | C | Other Ag–Ab | Result |
|---------|--------------|---------|-------------|---------------------|
| Present | Present | – | – | Agglutination |
| Present | Present | Present | – | Lysis |
| Present | Present | Present | Present | Inhibition of lysis |
| Present | – | Present | – | None of these |

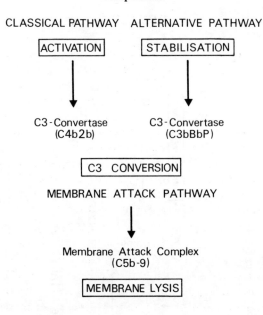

**Fig. 6.1** Pathways of complement activation. See Fig. 6.2 and text for greater detail.

via the **membrane attack pathway** with the production of lytic lesions.

## The classical pathway

The first step involves the generation of an enzyme — C1 esterase — following a complex interaction between the three subunits of the first complement component C1 (C1q, C1r and C1s). The C1q molecule resembles a bunch of tulips and the critical requirement for C1 activation is that at least two of the six 'flower heads' of the C1q molecule interact with the Cγ2 domain of two adjacent IgG molecules (Fig. 6.3) or two comparable complement activating sites in the Cγ3 domain of two adjacent subunits of a single pentameric IgM molecule. In either case, these critical requirements are only fulfilled when the immunoglobulin is in complexed or aggregated form and this prevents the inappropriate activation of C1 by un-complexed antibody.

The conformational change induced results in activation of C1r, which then activates C1s to form the esterase (C$\overline{1s}$). This enzyme acts on the next component in the sequence, C4, to yield a small

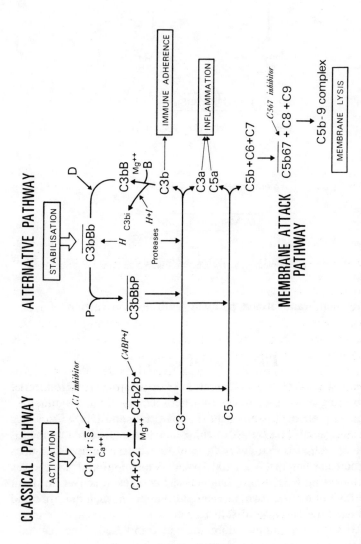

**Fig. 6.2** Overall plan of the **classical, alternative** and **membrane attack pathways** of complement activation. Individual components have numbers or capital letters, e.g. C4 or P. Lower case letters indicate complement fragments, e.g. C3b. A horizontal bar above a component indicates that it has become activated, e.g. C3b. Inhibitors are printed in italics. Ca$^{++}$ and Mg$^{++}$ indicate a requirement for divalent calcium or magnesium ions. See text for further description.

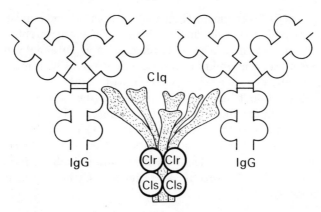

**Fig. 6.3** Interaction between the complement activating domains (Cγ2) of two adjacent IgG molecules and two of the subunits of Clq forming part of the Clq:r:s complex.

fragment C4a and a larger fragment C4b. The latter binds covalently to membranes in the immediate vicinity but with a short half-life. C4b binds C2 in the presence of magnesium ions, causing the C2 molecule to become susceptible to the action of C̄1̄s̄, which cleaves it to form a large C2b fragment and a small C2a fragment. C2b remains attached to C4b on the surface membrane and this complex, designated C̄4̄b̄2̄b̄, functions as a **C3 convertase** with a half-life of about 5 minutes at 37°C (Fig. 6.2).

The classical pathway can be activated by factors other than immunoglobulins, e.g. C-reactive protein, lipid A of bacterial endotoxins, polyanions, polycations and some virus membranes. Classical pathway activation is regulated by several inhibitors, e.g **C1 esterase inhibitor** (C1EI), which inactivates C̄1̄r̄ and C̄1̄s̄ as well as other serine esterases present in plasma. The combined activities of a **C4-binding protein** (C4BP) and **I** (an inhibitor which was previously called C3b inactivator because it also acts on C3b) limit the effect of C̄4̄b̄2̄b̄. C4BP accelerates the dissociation of C̄4̄b̄2̄b̄ and facilitates the cleavage of C4b by I.

## C3 conversion

This is the bulk reaction of the complement pathway during which several biological activities are generated. **C3 convertases** (C̄4̄b̄2̄b̄ or C̄3̄b̄B̄p̄P̄) cleave the α chain of C3 to give a small C3a fragment and a larger C3b fragment (Fig. 6.4). C3a causes degranulation of basophils and mast cells and is chemotactic for neutrophil polymorphs and for these reasons is referred to as an **anaphylatoxin**. C3b has a transient ability to form covalent bonds with membrane surfaces where it can act in concert with either of the two C3 convertases (C4b2b or C3bBbP) to trigger the membrane attack pathway by interacting with C5. C3b is inactivated by a combination of **factor I** and **factor H** which yields C3bi, which converts, after cleavage by trypsin-like enzymes, to C3d and C3c (Fig. 6.4). C3b also mediates the phenomenon of **immune adherence** by its ability to bind to **C3 receptors** (designated **CR1**) on polymorphs and monocytes.

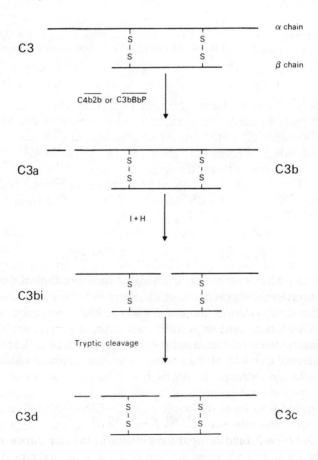

**Fig. 6.4** Sequential steps involved in C3 conversion.

# The alternative pathway

Another kind of C3 convertase can be formed by the stabilisation of a different set of proteins (but which includes C3b itself — a product of the classical pathway). Even in the absence of classical pathway activation, a degree of C3 conversion occurs due to spontaneous hydrolysis and this is enhanced by other proteases, e.g. plasmin, or other inflammatory products. This low-level or **tick-over** C3 conversion makes it possible for the alternative pathway to operate without activation of earlier components of the classical pathway. However, the complex which C3b forms with factor B in the presence of factor D, i.e. C3bBb, rapidly dissociates unless factors are present which can stabilise it. These factors include microbial polysaccharides such as endotoxin, zymosan, sialic acid-deficient erythrocytes, nephritic factor, aggregated forms of IgA and some subclasses of IgG (see Table 5.1).

The inhibitor H constantly acts to dissociate C3bBb but its affinity for C3b is considerably reduced when these stabilising factors are present. They offer a protected surface which shields C3bBb from the inhibitor and permits its interaction with another alternative pathway protein — properdin (P) — to form the stable **alternative pathway convertase** C3bBbP, which then acts on C3 (and C5) in equivalent fashion to C4b2b. Thus, the alternative pathway takes the form of a feedback loop that operates whenever C3b is formed and is sustained when factors are present to stabilise the assembly of its C3 convertase.

# The membrane attack pathway

When C3b binds to surfaces in close proximity to either of the two C3 convertases described above, the membrane attack pathway is set in train following cleavage of C5. However, only the first step, in which C5 is cleaved to form C5a and C5b, is enzymatic. C5a is the most potent of the anaphylatoxins and activates neutrophil polymorphs as well as mediating mast cell degranulation and neutrophil chemotaxis. Both C3a and C5a are inactivated by a carboxypeptidase. C5b has a labile binding site for cell membranes and binds C6 to form the stable complex C5b6 which then combines spontaneously with C7 to form C5b67. C5b67 has a short half-life but will bind to lipid membranes in the immediate vicinity and its promiscuous activity also damages cells that are not the primary focus for immunological attack — a phenomenon known as **reactive lysis**. C8 binds to this complex, which inserts itself into cell membranes. Incorporation of C9 into the complex causes further penetration of the lipid bilayer and results in osmotic lysis of the cell. The fully developed lytic lesion — known as the **membrane attack complex** — is a polymerised form of C5b9 and has the appearance of a plug or rivet in the electron microscope. This mechanism of cell disruption shows interesting similarities with cell-mediated cytotoxicity (see Chapter 9).

## Hereditary angio-oedema

C1 esterase inhibitor acts on various serine esterases including $\overline{C1r}$, $\overline{C1s}$, plasmin and kallikrein. A deficiency of this enzyme is associated with acute attacks of angio-oedema which usually follow minor trauma. C1 esterase inhibitor is important in controlling the action of plasmin and kallikrein in extravascular sites and in its absence the uncontrolled activation of C4 and C2 or of kininogen to bradykinin will occur with major effects on capillary permeability. This process does not cause effective C3 conversion as it mostly occurs in fluid phase without the generation of a stable membrane-bound C3 convertase.

## Nephritic factor

This is an IgG molecule with specificity for $\overline{C3bBb}$ and is present in the sera of most patients with mesangio-capillary glomerulonephritis or partial lipodystrophy. Its presence is usually associated with marked depletion of C3, evidence of alternative pathway activation and normal levels of C1, C4 and C2. As the reactivity of this antibody resides in its Fab portion it is regarded as an auto-antibody although purified nephritic factors have been shown to be of larger size than normal IgG and have an increased carbohydrate content. IgG antibodies reactive with the classical pathway C3 convertase $\overline{C4b2b}$ have been described in post-infective nephritis and systemic lupus although the link between infection and the development of these auto-antibodies is unclear.

## Solubilisation of immune complexes

Immune complexes have a greater tendency to aggregate if formed under conditions of complement depletion. The presence of an intact classical pathway retards precipitation and activation of the alternative pathway and the interposition of C3b into the antigen–antibody lattice is required for solubilisation to persist. The complement system thus has an important role in the processing of immune complexes to enable them to be cleared by the mononuclear phagocyte system which promotes the generation of B cell memory following the uptake of complexes in germinal centres. This role of complement may also explain the link between genetically determined complement deficiencies and a predisposition to immune complex disease.

## Complement polymorphisms

Heritable allotypic variation has been identified for many of the complement components (e.g. C4, C2, C3, C5, C6, C7, C8, factor B and factor D) and the loci for genes coding for C4, C2 and factor B are found in close association within the HLA complex (see Chapter 4). It is possible that some of the associations between certain HLA haplotypes and particular diseases may operate through functional differences in these variant complement proteins, particularly when there is little or no functional activity, e.g. as with the C4 null gene (see Chapter 15).

## Inherited deficiencies

Deficiencies of most of the individual complement components have been described and are briefly reviewed in Chapter 12.

## Further reading

Lachmann P.J. & Peters D.K. (1982) Complement. In Lachmann P.J. & Peters D.K. eds. *Clinical Aspects of Immunology*, 4th edn. Blackwell Scientific Publications, Oxford.

Schifferli J.A., Ng Y.C. & Peters D.K. (1986) The role of complement and its receptor in the elimination of immune complexes. *New England Journal of Medicine*, **315**, 488–95.

Whaley K. ed. (1987) *Complement in Health and Disease*. MTP Press, Lancaster.

# Chapter 7
# Phagocytes

Metchnikoff coined the terms 'macrophage' and 'microphage' for the two main varieties of phagocyte and believed that they had a more important role in protective immunity than Ehrlich's serum factors (i.e. immunoglobulins). However, in 1903 Almroth Wright demonstrated that the effector function of phagocytes is triggered by immunoglobulins — a similar state of affairs to that already described for the interaction between complement and immunoglobulin molecules. The clearance function of phagocytic cells — studied largely by the use of vital dyes — was emphasised in the definition of the 'reticulo-endothelial' system but in recent years this misleading term has been replaced by a return to a Metchnikovian division into **mononuclear phagocytes** and **neutrophil polymorphs**. Mononuclear phagocytes are given different names in different tissues (Table 7.1) and are often referred to, collectively, as the **mononuclear phagocyte system**. They differ in size and morphology from neutrophils and, in addition to their role as phagocytes, are also able to present antigen to T cells (see Chapter 2). When activated, they secrete many proteins.

**Table 7.1** Cells of the mononuclear phagocyte system.

| Cell | Tissue |
| --- | --- |
| Monocyte | Blood |
| Macrophage | Bone marrow, spleen, lymph node medulla, lung (alveolar and pleural), peritoneum |
| Langerhans cell | Skin |
| Veiled cell | Lymph |
| Interdigitating dendritic cell | Lymph node paracortex |
| Kupffer cell | Liver |
| Osteoclast | Bone |
| Type A cell | Synovium |
| Mesangial cell | Kidney |

# Macrophages

Macrophages are released from bone marrow as immature monocytes and mature in various tissue locations where they reside for weeks or years. They accumulate slowly at sites of infection, respond to a variety of stimuli (including lymphokines) and have considerable potential for synthesis, secretion and regeneration. **Azurophilic lysosomal granules**, which are more evident in monocytes than in mature macrophages, contain lysozyme, myeloperoxidase and acid hydrolases (Table 7.2). Macrophages also possess a non-specific esterase and produce various neutral proteases, e.g. collagenase, elastase and plasminogen activator. Other **secreted products** include many complement components (and inhibitors), coagulation factors, fibronectin, interleukin 1, interferon, colony stimulating factor (CSF) and prostaglandins, e.g. $PGE_2$ and $PGF_{2\alpha}$.

# Neutrophils

Polymorphonuclear neutrophil leucocytes mature and are stored in bone marrow and are released rapidly into the circulation in response to various stimuli, notably bacterial infection. Neutrophils are 'end-cells' and only remain in the circulation for a few hours before they migrate into tissues where they die within $1-2$ days.

**Table 7.2** Stored and secreted products of the macrophage

Contents of azurophilic lysosomal granules
  Myeloperoxidase
  Lysozyme
  Acid hydrolases
    e.g. $\beta$-glucuronidase, phosphatase

Other secreted products
  C1, C2, C3, C4, C5, B, D, properdin, I, H
  Neutral proteases
    e.g. collagenase, elastase, plasminogen activator
  Interleukin I
  Interferon
  Fibronectin, $\alpha2$ macroglobulin
  Coagulation factors
    e.g. tissue thromboplastin, V, VII, IX, X
  Prostaglandins
    e.g. $PGE_2$, $PGF_{2\alpha}$
  Colony stimulating factor (CSF)

**Table 7.3** Stored and secreted products of the neutrophil.

Contents of azurophilic granules
  Myeloperoxidase
  Lysozyme
  Acid hydrolases
    e.g. β-glucuronidase, phosphatase
  Cationic proteins

Contents of specific granules
  Lactoferrin
  Lysozyme
  Histaminase
  Transcobalamin

Other secreted products
  Leukotrienes
    $LTB_4$
    $LTC_4$, $LTD_4$, $LTE_4$ (SRS)
  Prostaglandins
    e.g. $PGE_2$

The functions of the neutrophil are mostly directed toward the killing and degradation of bacteria and are the major constituent of what, in the pre-antibiotic era, was known as 'laudable pus'. Their primary **azurophil lysosomal granules** contain several cationic proteins in addition to lysozyme, myeloperoxidase and acid hydrolases (Table 7.3). Unlike macrophages, they also possess **secondary specific granules** which contain lactoferrin (an iron-binding protein) as well as lysozyme, histaminase and transcobalamin II (a vitamin B12-binding protein). Neutrophil polymorphs are also a potent source of leukotrienes, e.g. $LTB_4$ — a chemotactic agent for polymorphs and monocytes — and $LTC_4$, $LTD_4$ and $LTE_4$ which together constitute **slow reacting substance** (SRS). They also produce prostaglandins, e.g. $PGE_2$, and a platelet activating factor (PAF).

# Common features of phagocyte responses

Both kinds of cell respond to infective stimuli with the following sequence of activities: chemotaxis, target recognition, ingestion, killing and degradation.

**Chemotaxis**

Phagocytes exhibit directed movement along concentration gradients of chemotactic agents, e.g. **anaphylatoxins** (C3a, C5a), **leukotriene B4**, lymphocyte-derived chemotactic factor (LDCF) and phospholipids and peptides derived from bacteria. Neutrophils respond rapidly to these inflammatory stimuli by marginating to the walls of small blood vessels, adhering to endothelial cells and exiting into sites of inflammation.

## Target recognition

Phagocytes can interact with targets hydrophobically or via specific sugar residues, e.g. mannose, for which they have receptors. However, target recognition is greatly enhanced when specific antibody of class IgG or C3b becomes fixed to the target surface. Both neutrophils and macrophages possess specific **Fc receptors** for IgG1 and IgG3. Human polymorphs have 20 times as many receptors as macrophages and these receptors are more scarce on the immature monocyte. Neutrophil polymorphs also possess receptors of lower affinity for the Fc of IgA (Table 7.4). Both cells have receptors for C3b (**CR1**) and C3bi (**CR3**) which mediate the **immune adherence** phenomenon. The effective binding of complexed IgG to Fc receptors on phagocytic cells is largely due to a co-operative effect between adjacent IgG molecules brought together in an immune complex or other aggregated form rather than the development of a conformational change in the immunoglobulin molecule with the expression of a new binding site. The C3 receptor, on the other hand, only reacts with the converted C3b or C3bi fragments. C3 receptors are particularly effective in promoting the attachment of phagocytes to targets whereas Fc receptor binding induces ingestion and phagocytosis.

## Ingestion

Phagocytosis is a form of localised endocytosis and the reverse of the exocytotic process by which mast cells degranulate. It is an

**Table 7.4** Fc receptors on macrophages, neutrophils and eosinophils.

|  | IgG1 | IgG2 | IgG3 | IgG4 | IgA1 | IgA2 | IgE |
|---|---|---|---|---|---|---|---|
| Macrophages | ++ | − | ++ | − | − | − | + |
| Neutrophils | ++ | + | ++ | + | + | + | − |
| Eosinophils | + | + | + | + | − | − | + |

energy-dependent process in which the plasma membrane gradually envelops the ingested particle and buds off the surface membrane internally to form a phagosome. This then fuses with lysosomal granules to form the **phagolysosome** in which many of the processes take place which kill and degrade the ingested material.

## Killing and degradation

Phagocytes contain both oxygen-independent and oxygen-dependent options for microbial attack (Table 7.5). For example, **lysozyme** hydrolyses the peptidoglycan of Gram-positive cell walls; the acidic pH present in the phagolysosome is detrimental to many micro-organisms; **acid hydrolases** are able to digest many of its constituent materials; **basic cationic proteins** are active against both Gram-positive and Gram-negative organisms but mostly at alkaline pH and **lactoferrin** has a bacteriostatic effect due to its ability to bind iron strongly. Macrophages also secrete neutral proteases, complement components, coagulation factors and interferon and are able to recruit further cells via interleukin 1 and colony stimulating factor.

Phagocytosis is accompanied by a burst of respiratory activity initiated by a membrane oxidase which reduces molecular oxygen to the **superoxide** anion $(O_2^-)$ (Fig. 7.1). Most of the respiratory activity takes place within the hexose monophosphate shunt which provides NADPH as a fuel for the reduction of molecular oxygen. This process, which is initiated at the cell surface, continues on the inner surface of the phagolysosome. Superoxide is converted to

**Table 7.5** Lytic mechanisms of the phagocyte.

Oxygen-independent
  Lysozyme
  Lysosomal products
    cationic proteins
    acid hydrolases
  Lactoferrin (bacteriostatic)
  Neutral proteases

Oxygen-dependent
  Hydrogen peroxide
  Singlet oxygen
  Hydroxyl radical
  Hypohalite

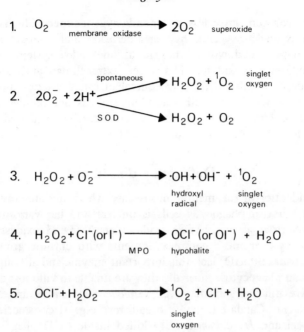

**Fig. 7.1** Sequential production of cytotoxic oxygen compounds in phagocytic cells. SOD = superoxide dismutase, MPO = myeloperoxidase.

**hydrogen peroxide** ($H_2O_2$) by spontaneous dismutation (predominantly at the cell surface) with the production of **singlet oxygen** $^1O_2$) or by the action of superoxide dismutase (SOD) (present intracellularly) giving rise to molecular oxygen. Singlet oxygen is a highly reactive and unstable molecular species which emits light as it returns to ground state. This process can be measured by the technique of chemiluminescence. Hydrogen peroxide and superoxide also interact to form another extremely reactive species — the **hydroxyl radical** ($\cdot OH$). A major source of microbicidal activity develops in the phagolysosome when hydrogen peroxide interacts with halide (Cl' in the neutrophil and I' in the macrophage) in the presence of **myeloperoxidase** (MPO) to form **hypohalite** and water. Hypohalite can then further react with hydrogen peroxide to form more singlet oxygen.

Thus it is clear that a variety of toxic materials are produced during the oxidative burst. Several processes limit the spread of these toxic effects. **Catalase**, largely present in peroxisomes, converts hydrogen peroxide to water and oxygen; **superoxide dismutase** converts singlet oxygen to hydrogen peroxide, and hydrogen peroxide is also broken down by the glutathione redox system involving glutathione peroxidase. The chief extracellular anti-oxidant is caeruloplasmin, which has an equivalent role to that of superoxide dismutase within the cell. Caeruloplasmin is one of several acute phase proteins whose synthesis is considerably increased by the liver following the release of interleukin 1.

## Deficiency disorders

The identity of the membrane oxidase which initiates the respiratory burst in phagocytic cells is unclear and has variously been characterised as an NADH oxidase, an NADPH oxidase and a flavin–cytochrome b complex. Patients with **chronic granulomatous disease** (CGD) lack this important enzyme and although their cells can phagocytose normally they are unable to kill most catalase-positive micro-organisms, e.g. *Staphylococcus aureus* and *Serratia marcescens*. Catalase-negative organisms, e.g. streptococci, pneumococci and *H. influenzae*, are killed inside CGD phagocytes as they produce their own hydrogen peroxide which, as it is not broken down by micro-organism derived catalase, is able to join forces with the phagocyte's myeloperoxidase to generate hypohalite and a cidal effect.

**C3 receptor deficiency** has been described in individuals whose phagocytes can mount a normal respiratory burst and show normal IgG-dependent phagocytosis (e.g. of *S. aureus*) but impaired complement-dependent phagocytosis (e.g. of opsonised yeast). The C3bi (CR3) receptor is deficient whereas the C3b receptor (CR1) is normal, indicating the importance of the former in promoting this form of phagocytosis. Both these deficiencies are discussed further in Chapter 12.

## Further reading

Leslie R.G.Q. (1984) Evaluation of phagocyte function. In Reeves W.G. ed. *Recent Developments in Clinical Immunology.* Elsevier, Amsterdam.
Van Furth R. (1985) *Mononuclear Phagocytes: Characteristics, Physiology and Function.* Martinus Nijhoff, Dordrecht.

# Chapter 8
# Mast cells, basophils and eosinophils

For almost a century, three other kinds of granulocyte, mast cells, basophils and eosinophils, have been distinguished by the differential staining characteristics of their granules. In mast cells and basophils this is due to the presence of an acidic proteoglycan; in eosinophils the characteristic granules contain several basic proteins. The basophil is a circulating cell whereas the mast cell is sessile and present throughout the body but chiefly in perivascular connective tissue, epithelia and lymph nodes. There is heterogeneity within the mast cell population and dye binding is considerably affected by the method of fixation as well as the individual stains used. In appropriately fixed sections, the granules of mucosal and connective tissue mast cells differ in their staining properties. Mucosal mast cells have some features in common with basophils (which contrast with connective tissue mast cells), i.e. they are smaller, short-lived, have chondroitin sulphate as acidic proteoglycan, are resistant to the inhibitory effect of sodium cromoglycate and require T cells for their growth and differentiation. Basophils have been identified in some forms of T cell-mediated immune responses, e.g. Jones—Mote or cutaneous basophil hypersensitivity (see Chapter 11), and the vagaries of fixation and staining techniques have probably caused them to be overlooked in other situations.

Mast cell **degranulation** has a general role in immunity by regulating the egress of inflammatory cells and molecules through endothelial tight junctions whenever a local inflammatory response is required to deal with a focus of infection. This increase in capillary permeability may be partly due to the contraction of endothelial cells similar to the effect on smooth muscle fibres elsewhere. It is likely that the remarkable variation in permeability that occurs in the post-capillary venule of the lymph node is regulated by a similar process of IgE or complement-mediated mast cell degranulation as mast cells are plentifully found at the corticomedullary junction of lymph nodes, when appropriate fixation and staining methods are used.

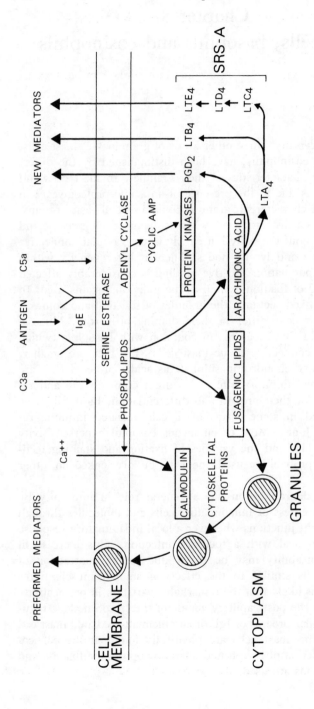

**Fig. 8.1** Processes involved in mast cell triggering and mediator release. See text for further details.

## Triggering of mast cells and basophils

Mast cells and basophils possess surface **Fc receptors** with a high affinity for **IgE**. Mast cells become activated either when surface-bound IgE molecules become cross-linked by antigen (or experimentally by anti-IgE) or following the local release of the **anaphylatoxins** C3a or C5a which have a direct effect on mast cell membranes. In either case, a complex series of events follows in which various membrane enzymes are activated, calcium ions enter the cell, and granules and their preformed mediator contents are released by exocytosis (Fig. 8.1). New mediators generated from arachidonic acid metabolism are released over a longer time-scale, traditionally referred to as **slow reacting substance** of anaphylaxis (SRS).

The initial step involves the activation of a serine esterase followed by the activation of methyl transferases acting on membrane phospholipids, on the one hand, and adenyl cyclase which generates an increase in intracellular cyclic AMP and protein kinase activity, on the other. Phospholipid methylation and the action of phospholipases are associated with three important events: the opening of membrane **calcium channels**, the generation of **fusagenic lipids** which encourage the fusion of perigranular and cell surface membranes and the production of a supply of arachidonic acid from which various newly synthesised mediators are derived. The activation of adenyl cyclase is critical for mediator release although its inhibition does not prevent phospholipid methylation. Once calcium enters the cell it is bound by calmodulin, which increases the activity of various enzymes (including protein kinases) and promotes the processes by which cytoskeletal proteins cause the contraction of microfilaments, leading to the extrusion of the granules and their contents. The anti-allergic drug **sodium cromoglycate** blocks mast cell degranulation and is thought to act by preventing the transmembrane influx of calcium ions.

## Mast cell mediators

The preformed mediators present within mast cell granules consist of **histamine**, eosinophil and neutrophil **chemotactic factors** (ECF and NCF), a proteoglycan, acid hydrolases (e.g. aryl sulphatase and β-glucuronidase) and neutral proteases (e.g. tryptase and chymase) (Table 8.1). Histamine is a small molecule which contracts smooth muscle and increases vascular permeability. It is present in mast

**Table 8.1** Stored and secreted products of the mast cell.

Preformed mediators
  Histamine
  Heparin proteoglycan
  Chemotactic factors (ECF and NCF)
  Acid hydrolases
    e.g. aryl sulphatase, β-glucuronidase
  Neutral proteases
    e.g. tryptase, chymase

Secondary mediators
  Leukotrienes
    $LTB_4$
    $LTC_4$, $LTD_4$, $LTE_4$ (SRS)
  Platelet activating factor (PAF)
  Prostaglandins
    e.g. $PGD_2$

cell granules as part of a protein complex with the proteoglycan **heparin**. Heparin is replaced by **chondroitin sulphate** in the basophil. Heparin is anticoagulant and anticomplementary and may have a role in promoting the diffusion of mast cell mediators despite activation of the coagulation pathway. The chemotactic factors released by mast cells not only attract other granulocytes but also increase the expression of their C3 receptors and have a stimulatory effect on the respiratory burst and the generation of oxygen-derived products.

SRS release takes place at a slower tempo than histamine release, the latter being a preformed mediator whereas the former has to be freshly synthesised. These 'secondary' mediators are lipid derivatives of **arachidonic acid** via two different pathways of metabolism under the control of cyclo-oxygenase and lipoxygenase enzymes (Figs 8.2 and 8.3). They include **SRS** (now known to consist of a combination of three different **leukotrienes**: $LTC_4$, $LTD_4$ and $LTE_4$), $LTB_4$ — a potent chemotactic agent, the prostaglandins $PGE_2$, $PGD_2$ and $PGF_{2\alpha}$ and platelet activating factor (PAF). The microsomal enzyme **cyclo-oxygenase** (also called prostaglandin synthetase) converts arachidonic acid to unstable intermediate cyclic endoperoxides ($PGG_2$ and $PGH_2$) which are then further metabolised to form stable prostaglandin mediators specific for each cell type. The predominant prostaglandin formed in mast cells is $PGD_2$ which contracts smooth muscle and is chemotactic for neutrophils. $PGE_2$ is produced in neutrophils, macrophages and lymphocytes

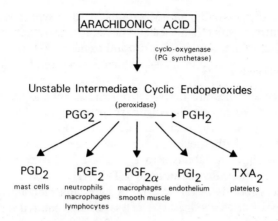

**Fig. 8.2** Products of the **cyclo-oxygenase** pathway and the cell types in which they are formed.

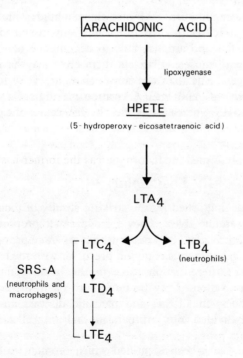

**Fig. 8.3** Products of the **lipoxygenase** pathway and the cell types in which they are formed.

and is a potent vasodilator. Macrophages also synthesise $PGF_{2\alpha}$ which contracts smooth muscle. Other stable prostaglandins produced by this pathway include thromboxane ($TXA_2$), formed in platelets, and prostacyclin ($PGI_2$), which is produced by endothelial cells.

The leukotrienes are derived from the metabolic oxidation of arachidonic acid by the **lipoxygenase** pathway in which the unstable 5-hydroperoxy-eicosatetraenoic acid (HPETE) is converted initially to the leukotriene $LTA_4$, which, depending on the cell concerned, either metabolises to $LTB_4$ (e.g. in neutrophils) or is converted by the SRS pathway to $LTC_4$, $LTD_4$ and $LTE_4$. This latter process occurs in various granulocytes and mononuclear cells and it is possible that at least two cell types are required for the full expression of leukotriene synthesis. SRS is a particularly potent constrictor of smooth muscle and a vasodilator. $PGD_2$ is the major arachidonic acid metabolite formed in connective tissue mast cells whereas $LTC_4$ production is prominent in mucosal mast cells and basophils.

**Platelet activating factors** (PAF) are phospholipids which cause calcium-dependent release of histamine and 5-hydroxytryptamine (5HT) from platelets and are also able to degranulate neutrophils and contract smooth muscle. Platelets themselves may have more of an immunological role than previously thought. They have Fc receptors for both IgG and IgE. Activation via the IgG receptor causes release of 5HT whereas triggering by IgE causes the generation of oxygen metabolites and a lytic effect on some parasites, e.g. schistosomes.

# Eosinophils

Eosinophils are distinguished by the striking affinity of their granules for acid or aniline dyes. They form a small proportion of peripheral blood leucocytes (1–5 per cent) but are more prevalent in tissues. They probably share a common precursor with the basophil and show a later differentiation stage in the blood comparable to macrophage activation. They become more plentiful (in blood and relevant tissues) in allergic and parasitic diseases and their functions can be divided into anti-parasite and anti-inflammatory activities.

Various factors have been identified which promote eosinophil proliferation and differentiation, e.g. colony stimulating factors, interleukin 2 and other eosinopoietic factors. Eosinophils also show a brisk chemotactic response to several materials liberated during the immune response, e.g. **ECF** (from mast cells), C5a and a T cell-derived factor. ECF and C5a display synergism in their chemotactic effects on eosinophils.

Eosinophils phagocytose poorly but degranulate promptly in the presence of chemotactic factors and when membrane bound IgG or IgE is cross-linked by antigen, i.e. exocytosis is more marked than endocytosis following triggering of their surface membrane, in contrast to the neutrophil. They have Fc receptors for both IgG and IgE isotypes (see Table 7.4), although the latter are of lower affinity than the IgE receptors on mast cells, and, like neutrophils, they also possess C3b receptors. They are able to form phagolysosomes following membrane triggering but this phenomenon is much less marked than in the neutrophil, and eosinophils display only limited proteolytic activity. Some of the contrasting features between mast cells, eosinophils and neutrophils are summarised in Table 8.2.

Eosinophils display an oxidative burst with generation of $H_2O_2$ and, probably, superoxide but it is uncertain whether they produce

**Table 8.2** Contrasting features of connective tissue mast cells, eosinophils and neutrophils.

|  | Mast cells | Eosinophils | Neutrophils |
|---|---|---|---|
| Lifespan | Long-lived | Long-lived | Short-lived |
| Dynamics | Sessile | Mobile | Mobile |
| Chemotactic response | − | +++ (ECF, C5a, T cell factor) | +++ (NCF, C5a) |
| Degranulation response (exocytosis) | +++ | +++ | + |
| Phagocytosis (endocytosis) | − | + | +++ |
| Lytic ability | − | +++ (basic proteins, O radicals) | +++ (lysosomal enzymes, O radicals) |
| Receptors for cell triggering | IgE C3a C5a | IgE IgG C3b | IgG IgA C3b |
| Biological role | Gatekeeper | Anti-helminth, anti-inflammatory | Anti-bacterial |

the other more lytic oxygen radicals found in the neutrophil (see Fig. 7.1). Eosinophil peroxidase (EPO) is different from myeloperoxidase (MPO) but may be able to work in concert with hydrogen peroxide and iodide or chloride ions to lyse some micro-organisms, e.g. *Trichinella*. However, the major source of lytic activity in the eosinophil is the basic or **cationic proteins** contained within the characteristic granules which are freely exocytosed during the degranulation response and are directly toxic to parasites, e.g. *schistosomes*, as well as to host cells.

## Eosinophil granules

The characteristic granules have a crystalloid core consisting largely of a **major basic protein** and a peripheral matrix containing other basic proteins, e.g. **eosinophil cationic protein** (ECP), and eosinophil-derived neurotoxin (EDN), as well as eosinophil peroxidase. Separate smaller granules contain aryl sulphatase and acid phosphatase. Eosinophil granules do not contain lysozyme. The exact location of other enzymes released by the cell, e.g. histaminase, β-glucuronidase and phospholipase D, is unclear. The protein which forms Charcot–Leyden crystals in various tissues and body fluids subjected to eosinophil degranulation is a lysophospholipase which resides in the plasma membrane of eosinophils (and basophils). Eosinophils also produce large amounts of platelet activating factor (PAF), leukotrienes, e.g. $LTB_4$ and $LTC_4$, and prostaglandin E2. Several of these eosinophil products have an inhibitory effect on mast cell mediators (Table 8.3) and it is for this reason that the

**Table 8.3** Interactions between mast cell and eosinophil products.

| Inflammatory mediators produced by mast cells | Inhibitory activities produced by eosinophils |
| --- | --- |
| Histamine | Histaminase<br>$PGE_2$ |
| Heparin | Major basic protein |
| SRS<br>LTB<br>$PGD_2$ | Aryl sulphatase<br>Peroxidase |
| PAF | Phospholipase |

eosinophil is regarded as having an anti-inflammatory role as well as destructive effects on parasites.

## Hypereosinophilic syndrome

The release of inflammatory mediators can have serious complications in patients with the **hypereosinophilic syndrome** (HES). These consist of endomyocardial fibrosis and thrombo-embolic disease, largely associated with the liberation of the toxic basic proteins and platelet activating factor, respectively.

## Further reading

Capron A. *et al.* (1986) From parasites to allergy: a second receptor for IgE. *Immunology Today*, 7, 15–18.

Jarrett E.E. & Haig D.M. (1984) Mucosal mast cells *in vivo* and *in vitro*. *Immunology Today*, 5, 115–19.

Parker C.W. (1984) Mediators: release and function. In Paul W.E. ed. *Fundamental Immunology*. Raven Press, New York.

Spry C. & Tai P.-C. (1984) Eosinophils in disease. *Journal of the Royal Society of Medicine*, 77, 152–5.

# Chapter 9
# Killer cells

Various cells of the immune system are able to inflict mortal damage on other living cells, e.g. bacteria, viruses, protozoa, the component cells of foreign grafts and even, in some circumstances, host tissues themselves. The ability of macrophages, neutrophils and eosinophils to release lysosomal enzymes, toxic basic proteins and lytic oxygen radicals has already been reviewed. Other cells, referred to here as killer cells, specialise in the lytic damage of target cells by events which take place within or upon their cell membranes, e.g. **T killer cells** $(T_k)$ and cells which currently go under a variety of names but which are most often referred to as **natural killer** (NK) cells.

## T killer cells $(T_k)$

This subset of T lymphocytes differentiates from cytotoxic precursor T cells $(T_{cp})$ following the release of interleukin 2 from T helper cells $(T_h)$. Until recently it was thought that killer activity coincided with the T8 subset of T lymphocytes but it is now clear that some T4-positive cells can also be cytotoxic (see p. 32 and Fig. 3.1). In each case, these cells bear a specialised antigen receptor which displays the phenomenon of dual recognition in which foreign, e.g. virus, determinants are recognised concomitantly with HLA glycoproteins on the target cell membrane. T8-positive cells recognise antigen with HLA class II whereas T4 cells bind to antigen associated with HLA class I.

Killer T cells have a key role in the lysis of host cells infected with budding viruses, i.e. those viruses which do not have a significant extracellular phase, and thus are not amenable to the effects of immunoglobulin working in conjunction with complement or phagocytes.

T cell killing occurs in three distinct phases:
**1 Recognition and adhesion.** Avid binding of target cell determinants by specific receptors on the $T_k$ cell lasts for a few minutes at 37°C. The effector cells need to be metabolically active (although

the target cells do not) and this event can be blocked by membrane-modifying agents, e.g. cytochalasin and local anaesthetics.

**2 Lethal hit**. This energy-independent step requires calcium ions and lasts about 10 min at 37°C. It is at this stage that changes in target cell membrane permeability are first detectable due to the insertion of hydrophobic tubular channels derived from the polymerisation of precursor materials present in the Golgi apparatus and cytoplasmic granules of the cytotoxic T cell.

**3 Osmotic lysis**. This stage lasts for at least 60 min during which the target cell dies due to the osmotic influx of water and rupture of the cell. Continued contact with the $T_k$ cell is not required. Neither of the last two phases are inhibitable by pharmacological agents.

$T_k$ cells can detach and recycle for further lytic events after inflicting a lethal hit on a target cell and recent work indicates that a $T_k$ cell can kill any other cell that binds to it, once it has been triggered by the recognition of a specific target. It is not yet clear what agency modulates the $T_k$ cell back to its resting state or whether it only survives for a short period of lytic activity but prostaglandins of the E series have an inhibitory effect on T cell killing. Soluble **lymphotoxins** are released by cytotoxic T cells but are of secondary importance to events taking place at the cell membrane as lysis can still occur when the production of these factors is inhibited.

This mechanism of target cell lysis, whereby a hydrophobic tubular structure is inserted into the target cell membrane, is very similar to that described for the lytic events induced by NK cells (see below) and also shows considerable similarity to the formation of the membrane attack complex (MAC) in the terminal pathway of complement activation (Chapter 6).

Examination in the electron microsope reveals the presence of granules in all cytotoxic lymphocytes. These contain lysosomal enzymes, e.g. acid phosphatase and aryl sulphatase, both of which are deposited at effector–target cell junctions although they do not contain materials characteristic of mast cells and macrophages, e.g. histamine and neutral proteases. Isolated granules have been shown to form cylindrical structures in the presence of calcium ions and study of the pores which they form has led to the characterisation of pore-forming proteins or **perforins**.

The size of the tubular structures formed during lymphocyte and complement-mediated cytotoxicity is significantly different and, although colloid osmotic lysis may be the final act in complement lysis, local damage with bulging and blebbing of target cell membranes suggests qualitative differences from the final events of $T_k$ and NK lysis. Oxidative pathways are unlikely to make a major contribution to $T_k$ and Nk lysis as they are absent in chronic granulomatous disease in which NK activity is normal and, conversely, are present in the Chediak—Higashi syndrome in which NK activity is deficient but oxidative pathways are preserved (see below).

## The 'null' or 'third cell' population

In human peripheral blood, T and B lymphocytes only account for about 75 per cent and 10 per cent, respectively, of mononuclear leucocytes. The residuum of $c$. 15 per cent of cells has often been referred to as the 'null' or 'third cell' population in view of their lack of T and B cell markers. Only a very small proportion of these null cells are monocytes and it is important to note that the term 'mononuclear' is a general descriptive term for all white cells possessing a single nuclear form and is not synonymous with the mononuclear phagocyte or monocyte, which is but one example of such a cell.

Non-phagocytic null cells have a number of characteristics which distinguish them from T and B lymphocytes and this has resulted in a confusing array of names and designations being given to them:

1 When B cell numbers were compared by counting the number of mononuclear cells bearing surface immunoglobulin at 4°C and 37°C, it was observed that a number of cells shed surface-bound Ig after washing and incubation at 37°C and thus were not true B cells. These have been referred to as L cells in view of the temperature-*labile* binding of IgG to their Fc receptors.

2 It was observed that some mononuclear cells were able to lyse target cells providing that IgG antibody specific for the target was present. This phenomenon of **antibody-dependent cell cytotoxicity** (ADCC) is largely attributed to members of the null cell population, which have also been referred to as K cells, although macrophages and eosinophils can also lyse targets in the presence of specific antibody of IgG class.

3 Studies of target-specific T cell cytotoxicity often give high levels of background cytotoxicity which is not target-specific and is attributable to contamination with non-T cells which are able to kill

in a less specific way and which have been referred to as **natural killer** (NK) cells.

4 Attention has focused on one or two large azurophilic granules which many of these null cells contain and this has led to their designation as **large granular lymphocytes** (LGL).

After more than a decade of confusion it is now clear that the characteristics denoted by the terms L, K, ADCC, NK and LGL all reside within the same cell population and for the present these cells will be referred to as LGL/NK cells.

## LGL/NK cells

The major properties of LGL/NK cells are set out in Table 9.1. These effector cells show spontaneous killing against various targets without the MHC restriction of T cells and are also able to kill a wide range of IgG-coated targets but lack the properties of classical macrophages, polymorphonuclear leucocytes or cytotoxic T cells. Their presence and activity is readily detectable in peripheral blood, to a lesser degree in the spleen and at a low level in lymph nodes, bone marrow and mucosa-associated lymphoid tissue (MALT). NK activity has been detected in the thymus but these cells are also present in athymic animals. T cell receptor gene studies have recently shown that NK cells possess rearranged genes for the β chain of the T cell receptor and thus it is most likely that the LGL/NK cell is a pre-thymic pre-T cell. Less mature forms of LGL/NK cells are positive for the CD 2, 3 and 8 T cell markers (see Table 3.1) and lose these as they acquire their distinctive granules and Fc receptors for IgG. There is also evidence that LGL/NK cells may have a suppressor role, e.g. in pregnancy, and the observation that suppressor T cells possess Fc receptors for IgG

**Table 9.1** Characteristics of LGL/NK cells.

| |
|---|
| Large azurophilic granules |
| Secondary lysosomes contain acid phosphatase |
| Absent peroxidase and non-specific esterase |
| Well-developed Golgi apparatus |
| Fc receptors for IgG |
| C3b receptors (CR3) |
| ADDC and NK activity |
| Non-T suppressors |
| Respond to IL-2 and interferon |

may well be explained on the basis of contamination with LGL/NK cells.

## Lytic mechanism

LGL/NK cells are non-phagocytic and non-adherent. Their azurophilic granules contain β-glucuronidase and are almost certainly the source of the lytic factors or **perforins** which polymerise to form tubular complexes and create pores in the target cell membrane and cause its lysis. These tubular complexes are similar to the complement-generated membrane attack complex. A chondroitin sulphate proteoglycan is also released from the granules during NK lysis and may act as a carrier or inhibitor of the lytic factor. LGL-NK cells possess a well-developed Golgi apparatus, which orientates towards the target cell during lysis, and vacuoles — probably equivalent to the lysosomal granules of monocytes and neutrophils — which contain acid phosphatase. These cells do not contain cytoplasmic peroxidase and are negative for non-specific esterase. However, they do have an oxidative burst and make plentiful superoxide although this seems to contribute very little to their lytic activity. This is borne out by the fact that patients with chronic granulomatous disease have an impaired oxidative burst but normal NK activity whereas patients with the Chediak–Higashi syndrome (and mutant Beige mice) have absent NK activity but normal oxidative metabolism. These deficiency disorders are discussed further in Chapter 12.

LGL/NK cells are activated by all three varieties of interferon (α, β and γ) and by interleukin 2. They secrete a variety of materials following target recognition, including interferon, interleukin 1, interleukin 2 and other growth factors and granule-derived lytic factors. They do not synthesise immunoglobulin.

LGL/NK cells are particularly effective at lysing tumour cells, virus-infected cells and cells of bone marrow origin. The specificity of their reactivity is still poorly understood but the determinants they recognise are high molecular weight glycoproteins and are probably closely related to class I HLA molecules. The fact that the lytic process can be triggered either by direct membrane contact or via surface-bound IgG makes an interesting comparison with mast cell triggering where the signal is transmitted either by cross-linking of surface-bound IgE or by a direct effect of C5a. Study of LGL/NK cell clones indicates that these cells show a degree of polyclonality although their specificity repertoire does not seem to be as extensive as that of the cytotoxic T cell. Nevertheless, the lesions induced by both kinds of cytotoxic cell are remarkably similar at the ultrastructural level.

## Further reading

Henkart P.A. (1985) Mechanism of lymphocyte-mediated cytotoxicity. *Annual Review of Immunology*, **3**, 31–58.
Tschopp J. & Conzelmann A. (1986) Proteoglycans in secretory granules of NK cells. *Immunology Today*, **7**, 135–6.

# IMMUNOPATHOLOGY AND
# TRANSPLANTATION

# Chapter 10
# Allergy and auto-immunity

The primary role of the immune system is to protect the host against a variety of pathogenic infections. However, it is almost notorious for its capacity to cause inflammatory damage to host tissues during the course of such infections and this chapter reviews the various ways in which the immune system causes pathological damage. This forms the basis of **immunopathology**.

## The host–pathogen interface

The complexity of the immune response and, in particular, the variety of effector mechanisms by which pathogens are destroyed are a reflection of the many diverse forms of pathogen that may confront it (see Chapter 1). Infectious diseases remain a major cause of illness and death throughout the world and Table 10.1 lists some of the more important infections prevalent today.

The balance is shifted in favour of the host when the pathogen becomes weakened or attenuated and chemotherapy greatly assists this process, when available. However, for infections which are a threat to life, the most satisfactory goal is that of prophylactic

**Table 10.1** Examples of major infections prevalent today.

| | |
|---|---|
| Metazoa | Filariasis |
| | Hookworm |
| | Schistosomiasis |
| Protozoa | Amoebiasis |
| | Malaria |
| | Trypanosomiasis |
| Bacteria | Tetanus |
| | Tuberculosis |
| | Typhoid Fever |
| Viruses | Hepatitis |
| | Measles |
| | Polio |

immunisation and several of the infections listed in Table 10.1 form part of the World Health Organisation's special programme for tropical disease research. The development of vaccines against some of the more successful and persistent parasites will, nevertheless, require considerable ingenuity and resources, for these pathogens have evolved their own ways of evading the attentions of the immune response (see p. 18).

## Allergy or hypersensitivity

Inflammation is a well-known consequence of infection and its classical signs of **rubor** (erythema), **tumor** (swelling), **calor** (heat) and **dolor** (pain) were described by Celsus *circa* AD 30. The identification of noxious materials produced by pathogens, e.g. diphtheria and cholera toxins, led to the general view that much of the pathology of infectious disease was due to the evils of the infecting organism whose ill effects the immune response was endeavouring to contain. However, much of the discomfort and disability is often a direct consequence of the activities of the immune response against the pathogen and this is well illustrated by studies performed with LCM virus.

If adult mice of a certain strain are inoculated with **lymphocytic choriomeningitis** (LCM) virus they develop fits and paralysis due to an acute encephalitis (Fig. 10.1). If inoculation is performed when the animals are newborn they do not become ill, even when reinoculated as adults, although they remain lifelong carriers of the virus. If adult animals are given a single dose of a cytotoxic drug — cyclophosphamide — shortly after the inoculation of LCM virus

**Table 10.2** Some infectious diseases or their complications in which immunologically-mediated tissue damage is a major feature.

| Disease | Infectious agent |
| --- | --- |
| Acute pneumonia | *Pneumococcus* |
| | *Staphylococcus* |
| | *Legionella* |
| Pulmonary tuberculosis | *M. tuberculosis* |
| Tuberculoid leprosy | *M. leprae* |
| Syphilis | *T. pallidum* |
| Serum hepatitis | Hepatitis B virus |
| Glomerulonephritis | *Streptococcus* |
| | *P. malariae* |
| Rheumatic fever | *Streptococcus* |

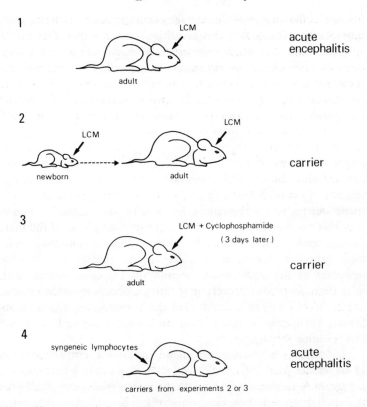

**Fig. 10.1** Experiments with LCM virus in mice. See text for further details.

they too suffer no ill effects and continue to harbour the virus. Either of these two 'carrier states' can be rapidly terminated by the administration of histocompatible lymphocytes from a normal animal (experiment 4, Fig. 10.1). These findings indicate that the severity of the tissue damage is governed by the vigour of the immune response rather than the continued presence of the virus. The former can be subverted by administering the virus before the animal is immunologically mature or eliminated by the adminis-tration of a drug which kills the specifically reactive cells of the immune response as they proliferate in response to the introduction of the virus.

There are many examples of infections in which there is good evi-dence for a major contribution by the immune response to the tissue damage which ensues, and some of these are listed in Table 10.2.

Massive inflammatory lung damage occurs in acute bacterial **pneumonia** and, even today, this condition carries a mortality rate of *c.* 10 per cent even when appropriate antibacterial agents are used. Several of the important organisms concerned, e.g. pneumococci, staphylococci and *Legionella*, possess subtle ways of evading the immune response (see p. 18). Much of the tissue destruction (caseation) seen in post-primary **pulmonary tuberculosis** is due to the intensity of the cell-mediated immune response to the *Mycobacterium*: the latter presents particular problems to the immune response because of its waxy coat and intracellular location. Infection with *Mycobacterium leprae* is also very difficult for the immune response to eradicate and individuals may show dramatic signs of tissue destruction (tuberculoid leprosy) or the immune response may become overwhelmed (lepromatous leprosy). Most of the tissue damage seen in secondary and tertiary **syphilis** is immunologically mediated. The severity of infective serum **hepatitis** is largely determined by the intensity of the immune response and acute infection of the throat with certain strains of β-haemolytic streptococci can be followed by inflammation of the heart and joints (**rheumatic fever**), basal ganglia (involuntary movements) and kidneys (acute **glomerulonephritis**).

Untoward responses of this kind have often been referred to as hypersensitivity or allergy and can also occur when vaccines are used. A vaccine against **respiratory syncytial virus** (RSV) was withdrawn when it was discovered that children who received it experienced a greater degree of lung damage (due to immune complex formation) when they subsequently contracted the natural infection. The first **measles** vaccine to be introduced was a heat-inactivated preparation but this gave rise to an unusually severe and atypical form of measles following natural infection and was withdrawn in favour of the current live attenuated vaccine which does not have this effect. The first descriptions of **anaphylaxis** and **serum sickness** followed exposure to inanimate material (jelly fish extract and horse serum, respectively) although these can also occur during infection (e.g. hydatid disease and viral hepatitis).

The term **allergy** is mostly used to refer to untoward responses to inanimate or non-pathogenic materials. Table 10.3 lists some of the more common offending agents. Immunological responses to materials of this kind can affect the skin (e.g. **eczema** and **dermatitis**), the lungs (e.g. **asthma** and **alveolitis**), and the gut (e.g. **coeliac disease** and malabsorption). However, there is marked variation in individual susceptibility to develop allergic responses

**Table 10.3** Some non-infective materials which can trigger allergic responses.

Plant pollens
Fungal proteins
Animal danders
House dust mite proteins
Insect stings
Food proteins
Drugs and chemicals
Metals, e.g. chromium, cobalt and nickel
Vaccines

and many of them fall within the general category of atopic disease, which is discussed further on p. 122.

Many kinds of disturbance which have been loosely attributed to 'allergy' have nothing to do with immunological responsiveness and the cardinal features of immune responses (i.e. specificity, memory, amplification and self-discrimination) should be reviewed (see Chapter 1) when attempting to categorise an adverse reaction as immunological or not. Favism is a condition in which haemolytic anaemia and jaundice follow the ingestion of broad beans and various drugs. This was thought to be an immunological phenomenon until a deficiency of glucose-6-phosphate dehydrogenase was identified within the red cell membrane of susceptible individuals. Another example is the adverse response to aspirin and some other drugs and chemicals experienced by a few patients with asthma. In both instances the lack of chemical specificity was always against an immunological explanation. A now classic confusion is that of the inappropriately termed 'total allergy syndrome' in which some individuals experiencing a variety of symptoms including dizziness and breathlessness following exposure to many different stimuli were considered to have an immunological problem. Most of the symptoms described are now known to be psychological in origin and mediated by hyperventilation and hypocapnia.

The mechanisms whereby tissue damage is produced during the immune response to infective or inanimate material are discussed further in Chapter 11.

## Auto-immunity

Experimental work suggests that the ability of the immune system to discriminate between self and non-self is achieved by (a) a process whereby self-reactive cells are deleted during development and (b) the inhibition or regulation of residual self-reactive cells by other cells which suppress them either specifically (e.g. suppressor T cells) or non-specifically (e.g. NK cells). Some T lymphocytes escape the censoring process in the thymus by which self-reactive cells are eliminated and **clonal inhibition** is therefore required in addition to **clonal deletion**. B lymphocytes, on the other hand, are not subjected to self-reactive censoring but do not receive a 'go' signal from self-reactive T cells unless the normal immunoregulatory mechanisms have broken down.

Ehrlich contemplated the prospect of unbridled autoreactivity with the term '*horror autotoxicus*' and the first intimation of the existence of human auto-immune disease was the identification of a red cell auto-antibody (haemolysin) in a haematological complication of syphilis (paroxysmal cold haemoglobinuria). Many diverse forms of auto-immune disease have been studied since then and these disorders form a major part of clinical immunological practice. Often there are pointers toward microbial and chemical agents having a triggering role and there is considerable individual variation in host susceptibility, which governs the severity and chronicity of these processes.

## Induction of auto-immune responses

The development of auto-immune disease is still one of the unsolved mysteries of immunology although various mechanisms have been proposed for its induction (Table 10.4). Some bypass the requirement for self-reactive T cells although, by definition, this only provides a means of generating auto-antibodies and does not

**Table 10.4**  Possible ways of inducing auto-immunity.

---

**Bypassing unreactive T cells**
    Polyclonal B cell stimulation
    Carrier effect

**Stimulating auto-reactive T cells**
    Molecular mimicry
    Anti-idiotype reactivity
    Impaired immunoregulation (e.g. $T_s$)
    Inappropriate class II HLA expression
    Release of sequestered antigen

---

generate autoreactive T cells. A number of agents, e.g. endotoxin and EB virus, act as **polyclonal B cell stimulators** and this is probably why auto-antibodies appear transiently during the course of infectious mononucleosis. The **carrier effect** (Fig. 10.2) enables autoreactive B cells to receive T cell help when a foreign determinant, e.g. drug or virus, becomes covalently linked to a self-determinant. The helper T cells that recognise the foreign determinant can then co-operate with self-reactive B cells to cause them to proliferate and produce auto-antibody. Various experimental examples of this phenomenon have been studied and this process is thought to underly the auto-immune haemolytic anaemia that develops following the administration of the drug α-methyldopa or during infection with *Mycoplasma pneumoniae*. These foreign materials have been shown to become intimately associated with the red cell membrane.

Other explanations require the activation of autoreactive T cells which are normally quiescent. **Molecular mimicry** concerns the coincidence by which a pathogenic organism will contain a chemical determinant which exactly mimics a component of self. This

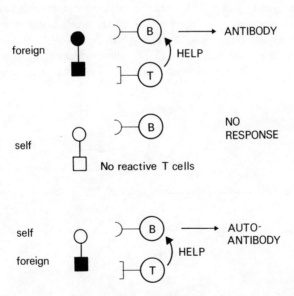

**Fig. 10.2** The **carrier effect** by which T cells reactive with foreign determinants can provide help for self-reactive B cells in the presence of covalently linked 'self' and 'foreign' determinants.

mechanism has been used to explain the presence in rheumatic fever of antibodies reactive with cardiac muscle which cross-react with a component of streptococci. There are likely to be many chance overlaps between foreignness and self and it seems likely that other requirements would have to be fulfilled before the normal process of immunoregulation is subverted.

There is now good evidence that, during the immune response to a foreign antigen (epitope), a second wave of antibodies appears which reacts with the **idiotype** of the initial antibody (see p. 53). The idiotype presents a complementary shape to that of the antigenic epitope and thus one would expect an anti-idiotype to show some similarity with the original epitope. It is likely, therefore, that a proportion of **anti-idiotype antibodies** will resemble determinants on the pathogen itself and can thus combine with host cell surface components, e.g. receptors, which have a particular affinity for foreign organisms, e.g. viruses (Fig. 10.3). Thus, some anti-idiotype antibodies will appear as 'auto-antibodies' and the same considerations apply to T cell reactivity. Anti-idiotype antibodies reactive with reovirus antibody have been shown to bind host cells and mimic or inhibit binding of the virus to these cells. The anti-receptor antibodies which occur in myasthenia gravis, thyroiditis and diabetes may arise in this way. This mechanism may help to explain why so many auto-antibodies are directed to structures with which viruses combine, e.g. DNA, ribonucleoprotein and various RNA fragments and enzymes, and why so many of the antibodies

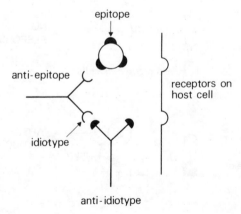

**Fig. 10.3** How anti-idiotype reactivity can manifest itself as auto-immunity. See text for further detail.

that develop during infection are not specific for the infecting organism.

The fact that some individuals and their families are inordinately prone to a variety of auto-immune disorders suggests that **impaired immunoregulation** may underly their susceptibility. The exact identity and role of suppressor T cells in man are ill-defined but various studies suggest that failure to control autoreactive helper T cells is of major importance in some auto-immune disorders. In particular, it may be critical in determining whether an auto-immune response is chronic or short-lived. Studies in mice demonstrate that red cell auto-antibodies can be readily induced by injecting the red cells of another species. The auto-immune response declines promptly in normal animals due to the presence of suppressor cells in contrast to animals prone to develop spontaneous auto-immune disease, e.g. the NZB/NZW hybrid mice.

Class II glycoproteins of the HLA system (see Chapter 4) are normally only expressed on antigen-presenting cells, e.g. macrophages and dendritic cells, and B lymphocytes. **Class II expression** has, however, been described on cells from tissues in which auto-immune disease has become established, e.g. thyrocytes in thyroiditis, pancreatic islets in type I diabetes and liver cells in biliary cirrhosis. It has been proposed that this stimulates autoreactive helper T cells to induce autoreactive cytotoxic T cells and B lymphocytes and ongoing auto-immune destruction. This could, conceivably, have survival value in enabling the host to eliminate persistent viruses within host cells but class II expression is a feature of most infective foci and sites of inflammatory damage and even though this may attract the attention of autoreactive helper T cells there is still a requirement for conventional antigen-presenting cells to generate interleukin 1 as the second signal for helper T cell stimulation. It is possible, therefore, that class II expression is a secondary rather than a primary phenomenon and may even have a role in inducing suppression as the immune response gets under way.

Lastly, self components that do not make contact with the cells of the immune system during development will not be regarded as 'self'. If material containing such components is released during adult life from a site in which it has been sequestered then a vigorous immune response will ensue and will be regarded as auto-immune. Lens protein and sperm antigens have been placed in this category to explain the development of sympathetic ophthalmia and mumps orchitis, respectively, although it is by no means clear how

many other kinds of auto-immune disease can be explained by the
**release of sequestered antigen.**

In most situations, it is likely that auto-immune disease arises
due to combinations of the processes listed in Table 10.4, e.g.
molecular mimicry is unlikely to wreak havoc in the absence of
other assistance such as class II expression, and immunoregulatory
impairment will become apparent when other forces, such as the
development of cross-reactive idiotypes, stimulate the production
of autoreactive specificities. Transient auto-immune phenomena are
extremely common in infectious disease and after the administration of some drugs and chemical agents. What is not clear is why
some patients present with severe and intractable auto-immune
disturbances which can be resistant to the most powerful immunosuppressive drugs.

Autoreactive T cells have recently been identified and isolated
from patients with auto-immune disease and studies using such
cell lines should provide valuable information concerning ways in
which the activity of these cells is regulated. The fact that they can
be obtained from animals who have recovered from an auto-
immune disease suggests that their active suppression is a normal
state of affairs.

**Table 10.5**   Auto-immune diseases and their typical auto-antigens.

**Organ-specific**

| | |
|---|---|
| Hashimoto's thyroiditis | Thyroglobulin |
| Graves' disease (thyrotoxicosis) | TSH[a] receptor |
| Pernicious anaemia | Intrinsic factor |
| Addison's disease | Zona glomerulosa of |
| | adrenal cortex |
| Type I (insulin-dependent) diabetes | Islet cells |
| Myasthenia gravis | ACh[b] receptor |
| Pemphigus | ICS[c] of epidermis |
| Pemphigoid | Epidermal BM[d] |
| Goodpasture's disease | Glomerular BM[d] |

**Systemic**

| | |
|---|---|
| Systemic lupus | Ds DNA[e] |
| Mixed connective tissue disease | Ribonucleoprotein |
| Systemic sclerosis | Nucleoli |
| Dermatomyositis | PM-1[f], JO-1[f] |
| Rheumatoid arthritis | IgG |

[a]TSH — thyroid stimulating hormone. [b]ACh — acetylcholine.
[c]ICS — intercellular substance. [d]BM — basement membrane.
[e]Ds DNA — double-stranded (native) DNA. [f]PM-1 and JO-1 are soluble
nucleoproteins.

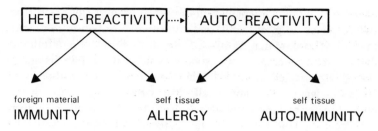

**Fig. 10.4** The spectrum of heteroreactive and autoreactive tissue damage.

The subdued but specific ability of the immune system to recognise self components is undoubtedly an important attribute, e.g. recognition of self HLA glycoproteins and recognition of self idiotypes, and is in keeping with the specialisation of the immune system from innate properties of intercellular recognition. Thus, autoreactivity may have greater physiological importance than was at first thought and should only be considered as untoward when expressed as the destructive lesions of auto-immune disease.

Some of the more common auto-immune diseases are listed in Table 10.5 in conjunction with the specificity of the auto-antibodies that characterise them. In some instances these antibodies have pathological effects, e.g. the anti-receptor antibodies of Graves' disease and myasthenia gravis. In others, tissue damage is largely due to the activities of T cells. In either case, the presence of auto-antibodies in the circulation is of considerable value in the serological investigation of these diseases and this is achieved by using the techniques described in Chapter 5.

## Pathways to immunological tissue damage

There are thus two main pathways by which immunological tissue damage may arise: that which follows responses which are formally directed toward foreign material, i.e. **heteroreactivity**, and responses direct at self components, i.e. **autoreactivity** (Fig. 10.4). In the former situation, the inflammatory effects of the immune response on foreign material fall within the definition of **immunity** whereas the 'bystander' effects on self tissue are referrred to as **allergy** or **hypersensitivity**. Autoreactivity can also lead to secondary bystander effects on self tissues which are not under specific attack although there is probably little point in attempting to distinguish between **auto-immunity** *per se* and hypersensitivity effects occurring as a non-specific sequel.

Although there are many well-described examples of heteroreactive responses (e.g. antiviral) and autoreactive responses (e.g. antithyroid) it is clear that most — if not all — forms of autoimmune disease are triggered by a response which, at least in its initial stages, is directed toward foreign material, be it pathogen or chemical agent. It is not at all clear why autoreactivity should predominate in some immune responses more than others but, as time goes by, the role of foreign determinants on pathogens (or other kinds of foreign material) is being incriminated in an increasing number of auto-immune diseases. Recent examples include infection with *Trypanosoma cruzi* and auto-immunity to heart muscle and Coxsackie virus and auto-immunity to pancreatic islets. If an infection is at all prolonged then it is probably unusual to find no evidence of autoreactivity whatsoever and it is interesting to speculate that if the *Treponema pallidum* had not been identified as the microbial cause of syphilis early on then much of the pathology present in secondary and tertiary syphilis (which includes the development of various kinds of autoreactivity) might well have been regarded as being due to auto-immunity.

## Further reading

Britten V. & Hughes H.P.A. (1986) Immunological recognition of altered cell surfaces in infection and disease. *Clinics in Immunology and Allergy*, **6**, No. 1.

Coombs R.R.A., Smith C.E.G. & Lachmann P.J. (1975) The allergic reactions as factors determining and influencing microbial pathogenicity. In Gell P.G.H., Coombs R.R.A. & Lachmann P.J. eds. *Clinical Aspects of Immunity*, 3rd edn. Blackwell Scientific Publications, Oxford.

Lessof M.H. (ed.) (1984) *Allergy: Immunological and Clinical Aspects*. Wiley, Chichester.

Mims C.A. (1982) *The Pathogenesis of Infectious Disease*, 2nd edn. Academic Press, London.

Plotz P.H. (1983) Auto-antibodies as anti-idiotype antibodies to antiviral antibodies. *Lancet*, **ii**, 824–6.

Rose N.R. & Mackay J.R. eds. (1985) *The Auto-immune Diseases*. Academic Press, London.

# Chapter 11
# Mechanisms of immunological tissue damage

Whatever the primary cause of a particular immunopathological disorder may be, the mechanisms by which host tissues become damaged belong to four main categories:

1 **Reaginic** or **anaphylactic**.
2 **Cell** or **membrane-reactive**.
3 **Immune complex**.
4 **Cell-mediated**.

This classification was originally developed by Coombs and Gell and grew out of the contrasting features of 'immediate' and 'delayed' forms of hypersensitivity. In Table 11.1 the physiological role of each mechanism is contrasted with pathological examples of heteroreactive and autoreactive tissue damage. Figure 11.1 illustrates these processes diagramatically.

## Reaginic mechanism

The reaginic or anaphylactic mechanism refers to the events which follow combination of antigen with IgE molecules specific for it upon the surface of mast cells. This involves the release of various mediators, e.g. histamine, leukotrienes (SRS), chemotactic factors (ECF-A and NCF-A) and platelet activating factor (PAF), which induce smooth muscle contraction and increase capillary permeability (reviewed in Chapter 8). The physiological value of this process has its origins in anti-parasite immunity in which increased vascular permeability promotes the extravascular recruitment of immunological components, e.g. IgG, neutrophils, eosinophils and monocytes, which can then act in concert to inflict damage upon the parasite by various forms of lysis. Smooth muscle contraction assists the process and, if it occurs in the gut, can lead to expulsion of the parasite.

Acute **anaphylaxis** is the systemic manifestation of this form of tissue damage and manifests itself as pallor, nausea, hypotension, itching, wheezing, cyanosis, abdominal pain, urticaria and loss of consciousness, all of which can develop over a remarkably short period of time, e.g. 5–10 minutes. In a susceptible individual, it

**Table 11.1** Mechanisms and examples of the four main categories of tissue damage.

| Mechanism | Physiology | Pathology | |
| --- | --- | --- | --- |
| | | Heteroreactive | Autoreactive |
| **Reaginic** | Extravascular recruitment of immunological components | Anaphylaxis Allergic asthma Allergic rhinitis | ? |
| | Parasite expulsion | | |
| **Cell or membrane-reactive** | Lysis of pathogens by extracellular or intracellular events | Incompatible blood transfusion | Haemolytic anaemia Thrombocytopenia |
| | | Haemolytic disease of the newborn | Pemphigoid Goodpasture's disease |
| | | Hyperacute graft rejection. | Myasthenia gravis[a] Thyrotoxicosis[a] |
| **Immune complex** | Neutralisation of pathogen-derived factors, e.g. toxins | Local | |
| | | Arthus reaction Dermatitis herpetiformis | Rheumatoid arthritis |
| | Transport of antigen to germinal centres | Allergic alveolitis Glomerulonephritis | |
| | | Systemic | |
| | | Serum sickness | Systemic lupus |
| | | Widespread vasculitis | Widespread vasculitis |
| **Cell-mediated** | Defence against intracellular parasites | Tuberculosis Leprosy Contact dermatitis Graft rejection | Thyroiditis Adrenalitis Pernicious anaemia Diabetes |

[a]The receptor antibodies present in these two conditions have inhibitory or stimulatory effects on the respective receptors rather than complement-mediated lysis.

can follow inoculation by a stinging insect, parenteral administration of an antibiotic, e.g. penicillin, or rupture of a hydatid cyst with release of antigen. Otherwise, pathological effects usually arise as a consequence of IgE production to inhaled or ingested antigens, e.g. pollens, animal danders and foods, and which, in affected

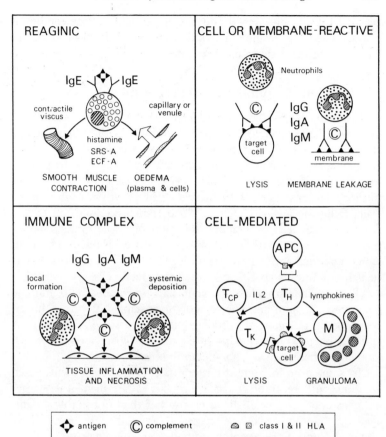

Fig. 11.1 **Mechanisms of immunological tissue damage**. SRS-A = slow reacting substance of anaphylaxis (consisting of leukotrienes LTC$_4$, LTD$_4$ and LTE$_4$). ECF-A = eosinophil chemotactic factor of anaphylaxis. APC = antigen-presenting cell. T$_{cp}$ = cytotoxic precursor T cell. T$_h$ = T helper cell. T$_k$ = killer T cell. M = macrophage. IL2 = interleukin 2. See text for further information.

individuals, overshadows any previous preoccupation with anti-parasite responses. Reaginic responses express themselves as extrinsic asthma in the lungs, allergic rhinitis in the nose and allergic conjunctivitis in the eyes, and other disorders affecting the gut, skin and kidneys fall within the general group of **atopic diseases** (see p. 122).

There are no well-documented examples of autoreactivity mediated by a reaginic mechanism but it is possible that an autoreactive IgE response could underlie one or other of the conditions characterised by eosinophilia and increased IgE production for which no primary cause has been identified.

## Cell or membrane-reactive mechanism

Cell or membrane-reactive tissue damage occurs when specific antibody (of classes IgG, IgA or IgM) combines with antigen on the surface of a cell or basement membrane and which is then able to activate complement and polymorphonuclear leucocytes. Its physiological role is the lysis of pathogens by these extracellular or intracellular processes. Their activity can prove disastrous, however, following an incompatible blood transfusion and during the antibody-mediated 'hyperacute' rejection of tissue grafts. Similar processes are involved in haemolytic disease of the newborn in which maternal antibody reacts with paternal blood group antigens (usually of Rhesus specificity) present on fetal cells.

This mechanism plays a major part in various auto-immune disorders, e.g. auto-immune haemolytic anaemia, idiopathic thrombocytopenic purpura, the bullous skin diseases (e.g. pemphigus and pemphigoid) and Goodpasture's disease (characterised by anti-glomerular basement membrane antibodies).

In some auto-immune disorders, antibodies are present which combine with receptors on cell surfaces rather than other target antigens and have metabolic effects rather than causing lytic damage, e.g. anti-acetylcholine receptor antibodies in myasthenia gravis and anti-TSH receptor antibodies in thyrotoxicosis.

## Immune complex mechanism

Immune complex-mediated tissue damage is probably the commonest form of all and occurs when soluble antigen combines with soluble antibody. In other words, this form of tissue damage is not confined to the surfaces of cells and can occur locally in a particular tissue or systemically via the circulation. As with the previous mechanism its inflammatory effects follow the activation of complement and phagocytic cells by immunoglobulins of classes IgG, IgA or IgM.

The combination of antibody with microbial toxins and other pathogen-derived factors has an important physiological role in neutralising their effects and antibody is also of critical importance in transporting antigen to germinal centres in lymphoid tissues to stimulate the recruitment and proliferation of B lymphocytes (see Chapter 3). If local concentrations of antigen become great then an excess of immune complexes will form followed by local tissue damage. This was originally described in the skin as the **Arthus** phenomenon following the repeated injection of heterologous serum. A contemporary example is farmer's lung in which the repeated inhalation of a provoking antigen gives rise to an allergic alveolitis. If excessive amounts of antigen occur in the circulation then immune complexes may deposit systemically. This was originally described in the form of **serum sickness** in which a rash, fever, arthritis and glomerulonephritis followed the injection of antidiphtheria horse serum. Similar reactions can follow the administration of drugs and during or following various infections. Immune complex-mediated damage is the basis of post-streptococcal glomerulonephritis, dermatitis herpetiformis, Henoch–Schonlein purpura and other forms of **widespread vasculitis**. Serum sickness-like features which occur in the early phase of viral hepatitis are also due to immune complex formation. This mechanism of damage is also seen in various auto-immune disorders, e.g. locally in joints in rheumatoid arthritis and in many organs in systemic lupus erythematosus.

## Cell-mediated mechanism

The cell-mediated mechanism is independent of antibody and occurs when T lymphocytes combine with cell surface antigens. The T cells recruit and activate monocytes and other T lymphocytes (including the precursors of cytotoxic T cells) and generate a powerful inflammatory response with lysis of the target cells. Physiologically, T killer cells are of particular importance in protection against intracellular parasites, e.g. mycobacteria and budding viruses. This mechanism of tissue damage is prominent in post-primary tuberculosis, leprosy and contact dermatitis and is the more usual means by which foreign grafts are rejected.

The cell-mediated mechanism is one of the slowest to develop and is often referred to as delayed hypersensitivity. The classical cutaneous reaction is usually evident within 24–48 hours but granuloma formation takes at least 14 days. Jones–Mote or cutaneous basophil hypersensitivity is a variant in which the cellular infiltrate contains many basophils and takes 7–10 days to develop, usually in response to soluble antigen. However, basophils and/or mast cells can be found in classical cell-mediated reactions if the necessary methods of fixation and staining are employed (see p. 81). The organ-specific group of auto-immune diseases, e.g. thyroiditis, adrenalitis, pernicious anaemia and type I diabetes, are all characterised by lymphocytic infiltration and lysis of hormone-producting cells and, recently, T cell clones have been derived from such patients which are reactive with organ-specific targets.

## Antibody-dependent cell cytotoxicity

Each of the four mechanisms described above require *either* specific antibody *or* T cells for their generation. There is another form of tissue damage which requires the co-operation of both antibody and lymphocyte-like cells, i.e. antibody-dependent cell cytotoxicity (ADCC). Various studies have demonstrated that combinations of IgG antibody and lymphocytes, IgG antibody and monocytes, IgE antibody and monocytes, and IgG antibody and eosinophils are each able to lyse target cells for which the antibody has specificity. Some of these events have been alluded to in the preceding discussion concerning the physiological role of the reaginic mechanism. However, it is not yet clear how important this group of mechanisms is in human immunopathology. Natural killer (NK) cells are also able to lyse target cells and do not require the presence of specific antibody. As discussed in Chapter 9, these cells overlap with lymphocyte-like cells that mediate ADCC and the role of NK cells in human immunopathology is, as yet, poorly understood.

These different mechanisms have been contrasted with each other for simplicity but it is not uncommon for more than one mechanism to coexist in a particular disease, e.g. injections of immunogenic material can give rise to anaphylactic and serum sickness-like reactions and both antibody-mediated and cell-mediated mechanisms have been identified in auto-immune thyroid disease. Recently, attention has focused on the role of immune complex formation in the lung in allergic asthma (in addition to the reaginic mechanism) (see p. 117). Unravelling the respective importance of these different processes in particular diseases is one of the challenges of clinical immunology and more detailed information will be found in postgraduate texts.

## Clinical examples

The mechanisms already discussed and their clinical effects are usefully contrasted by taking examples of immunologically mediated tissue damage occurring in the lung (Fig. 11.2). **Extrinsic allergic asthma** typifies the reaginic mechanism as exacerbations of this condition are induced when inhaled antigen makes contact with specific IgE on the surface of mucosal and submucosal mast cells, causing their degranulation and release of inflammatory mediators. These cause contraction of bronchial smooth muscle and a degree of bronchial oedema. Both processes cause narrowing of the airways and intermittent airways obstruction is the hallmark of this condition in contrast to chronic bronchitis and emphysema in which airways obstruction persists.

Maximal reduction in airflow occurs within 10 to 20 minutes of bronchial challenge with the relevant antigen. A similar latency of response is observed when prick tests are performed in the skin of susceptible subjects. This is in keeping with the earlier description of **immediate hypersensitivity** for the reaginic mechanism. However, a significant proportion of patients with extrinsic asthma show a second and more prolonged fall in airways obstruction several hours after inhalation of antigen. These changes are mediated by IgG, complement and neutrophils and thus involve an immune complex mechanism. This helps to explain why nocturnal asthma can be troublesome after daytime exposure.

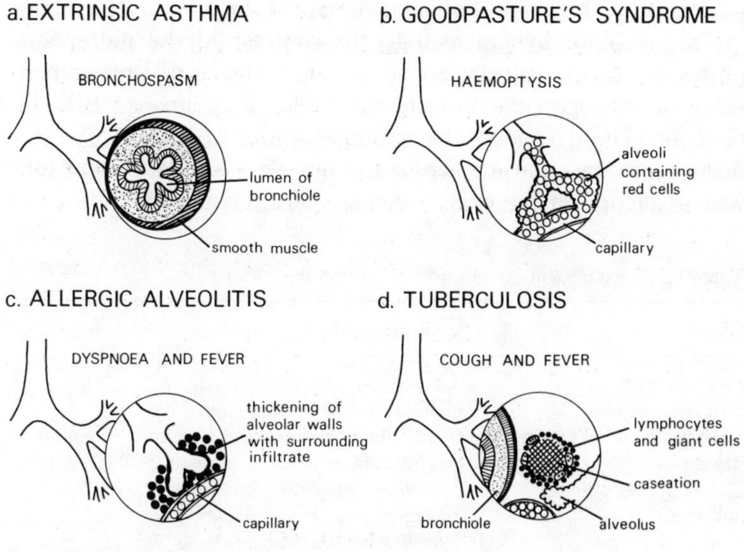

**Fig. 11.2** Examples of the four main types of immunological tissue damage occurring in the lung. See text for description.

A pulmonary example of the cell or membrane-reactive mechanism is **Goodpasture's syndrome** (Fig. 11.2b) in which auto-antibodies react with an antigen present in both glomerular and pulmonary basement membranes, giving rise to acute proliferative glomerulonephritis and parenchymal lung damage with bleeding from the lungs (haemoptysis); this condition is also referred to as lung purpura with nephritis. Damage to the basement membrane follows attachment of IgG antibody and activation of complement and phagocytic cells, culminating in the leakage of blood across it. Little is known about the cause of this condition although epidemiological evidence points to exposure to petrochemicals which, in susceptible subjects of HLA-DR2 phenotype (Table 4.1), is followed by the development of antibasement membrane antibodies.

Immune complex-mediated damage is exemplified by **extrinsic allergic alveolitis** in which IgG antibody is produced with specificity for inhaled antigen (Fig. 11.2c). The classical example is farmer's lung in which the antigen is a component of spores found in mouldy hay. IgG antibody complexes with antigen across the alveolar–capillary membrane, followed by complement fixation and activation of neutrophils. Clinically, this is manifest as breathlessness (dyspnoea), cough and fever occurring several hours after challenge and a similar latency is observed when skin tests are performed with the appropriate material. This led to the designation of **intermediate hypersensitivity** in contrast to the more rapid immediate form. Allergic alveolitis can follow exposure to many kinds of environmental antigen and Table 11.2 contains a brief list of them. The dyspnoea which follows acute exposure is due to a decrease in gas transfer across the alveolar–capillary membrane with reduction in the oxygen content of arterial blood. Wheezing

**Table 11.2** Example of extrinsic allergic alveolitis.

| Disease | Antigenic material |
| --- | --- |
| Farmer's lung | *Micropolyspora faeni* (mouldy hay) |
| Bird fancier's lung | Avian proteins (bird droppings) |
| Mushroom worker's lung | Thermophilic actinomycetes (mushroom compost) |
| Bagassosis | Thermophilic actinomycetes (mouldy sugar cane) |
| Cheese worker's lung | *Penicillium caseii* (mouldy cheese) |
| Suberosis | *Penicillium frequentans* (mouldy cork) |
| Malt worker's disease | *Aspergillus clavatus* (mouldy barley) |
| Ventilator pneumonitis | Thermophilic actinomycetes (humidifiers/air conditioners) |

or airways obstruction is not a feature of this condition. The proportions of inspired air to perfused blood present in different parts of the lung vary largely due to the effects of gravity on the circulation. In the upright position, the ventilation/perfusion ratio is high in the upper lobes of the lung and low in the lower lobes. Thus the changes of extrinsic allergic alveolitis are more commonly seen in the upper lobes whereas those of the intrinsic form are more commonly found in the lower zones.

**Intrinsic (cryptogenic) alveolitis** arises as a consequence of the deposition of blood-borne immune complexes in the pulmonary circulation, where they also cause complement and phagocyte activation within the alveolar–capillary membrane. This condition has a more insidious onset without evidence of acute exacerbation but produces similar effects on gas transfer. This condition often occurs in association with other auto-immune diseases, e.g. rheumatoid arthritis.

**Pulmonary tuberculosis** and **sarcoidosis** are examples of cell-mediated pulmonary damage. The former follows the inhalation of *Mycobacterium tuberculosis* and usually occurs in the upper lobes, whereas sarcoidosis — the cause of which is still unknown — is usually a more diffuse condition. Primary exposure to *M. tuberculosis* causes a small peripheral focus of infection (the **Ghon** focus) but with associated enlargement of the lymph nodes at the root of the lung. The primary focus usually heals without symptoms developing and it is only following subsequent (in this context usually referred to as 'post-primary') infection that severe damage to parenchymal pulmonary tissue develops in the upper zones of the lung (Fig. 11.2d). These changes follow activation of various subpopulations of T lymphocytes and the recruitment of macrophages as they respond vigorously to the re-introduced *Mycobacterium*. The involvement and recruitment of both lymphocytes and macrophages is probably why the tempo of this mechanism is the slowest of all and is often referred to as **delayed hypersensitivity**. An equivalent reaction takes place in the skin when sensitised subjects receive an intradermal injection of a mycobacterial extract as in the Heaf, Mantoux or Tine tests. A positive response is characterised by erythema, induration and itching occurring maximally 24–48 hours after challenge.

The intensity of the inflammatory response is such that, in the centre of a lesion, lung tissue is replace by cheese-like 'caseous' material often with the formation of cavities, which eventually become sealed off by fibrosis and calcification. It was only follow-

ing the introduction of effective anti-tuberculous drugs that this
condition (previously called 'consumption') lost much of its notor-
iety. Nevertheless, the efficacy of some of the more successful
agents, e.g. rifampicin, is due, at least in part, to an immunosuppressive effect. A similar pathology occurs in pulmonary sarcoidosis
except that infecting micro-organisms cannot be detected. It has
been argued that this is a response to an as yet unidentified pathogen
although an auto-immune aetiology is also a possibility.

The skin and kidneys are also involved in immunopathological
disorders and Fig. 11.3 contrasts examples of membrane-reactive
and immune complex damage in these two organs. The bullous or
blistering skin diseases, on the one hand, and various forms of
glomerulonephritis, on the other, demonstrate how relatively subtle
variations in the mechanism and locus of an immunopathological
disorder can produce major differences in clinical effects. **Pemphigus**
and **pemphigoid** are both caused by circulating auto-antibody

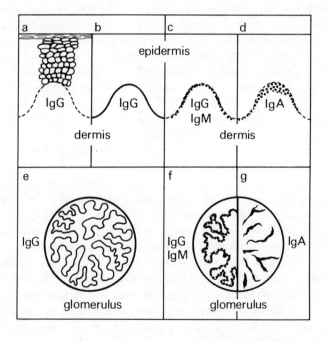

**Fig. 11.3** Examples of immunological tissue damage in skin (a–d) and kidney
(e–g): a — pemphigus, b — pemphigoid, c — systemic lupus (SLE), d —
dermatitis herpetiformis, e — Goodpasture's disease, f — systemic lupus (SLE), and
g — Berger's disease (IgA nephropathy).

reactive with cutaneous antigen. In the former the antigen forms part of the intercellular substance (ICS) of the epidermis and the interaction of IgG auto-antibody with it gives a typical 'chicken wire' pattern of staining on immunofluorescent examination of the skin (Fig. 11.3a). Complement fixation and disruption of the ICS leads to intra-epidermal blister formation. In pemphigoid, the antigen is a component of the epidermal basement membrane and immunofluorescent examination for IgG shows linear staining of this structure (Fig. 11.3b). Subepidermal blister formation follows complement activation at that site. **Dermatitis herpetiformis** is a bullous disorder in which IgA-containing immune complexes deposit in the papillary capillaries (Fig. 11.3d). These activate the alternative complement pathway in the dermal papillae and cause subepidermal blister formation. In **systemic lupus erythematosus** (SLE) IgG-containing immune complexes are found beneath the basement membrane of the epidermis (Fig. 11.3c) but although this may be associated with an erythematous rash this does not cause blisters to form.

In **Goodpasture's disease** auto-antibody to the glomerular basement membrane (GBM) can be detected by the presence of diffuse linear staining of the GBM on immunofluorescent examination (Fig. 11.3e). It usually causes an acute proliferative glomerulonephritis with reduced urine production (oliguria), blood in the urine (haematuria) and failure of the clearance function of the kidney (uraemia). Complement activation and infiltration by neutrophil polymorphs are pronounced features of this condition. Immune complex-mediated damage to the glomerulus takes many forms. Diffuse granular deposition of immune complexes containing most classes of immunoglobulin occurs in **SLE** (Fig. 11.3f) and thickening of the basement membrane as well as some degree of proliferative change is usually found in association with marked protein loss in the urine (proteinuria) and uraemia. In **IgA nephropathy** (Berger's disease), IgA-containing complexes preferentially localise to the mesangium of the glomerulus with relative sparing of the basement membrane, giving a radial pattern of deposition (Fig. 11.3g). The clinical features may range from haematuria and proteinuria to no clinical disturbance whatsoever. In some forms of immune complex deposition in the kidney, e.g. **membranous glomerulonephritis**, complexes localise in a subendothelial position where they are least able to recruit neutrophil polymorphs but give rise to considerable thickening of the basement membrane and marked proteinuria.

These examples have been selected to illustrate different patterns of immunologically mediated tissue damage in selected organs. More detailed descriptions of these and other disorders will be found in postgraduate texts.

# Atopic disease

Atopic disorders form a significant part of human immunopathology in the Western world, occurring in at least 5 per cent of individuals. The **atopic trait** can be defined as the spontaneous tendency for an individual to produce high levels of IgE reacting with one or more common antigens in association with antigen-provoked disorders in which a reaginic mechanism can be identified. Table 11.3 lists some of the more important conditions in which there is good evidence for the involvement of IgE antibody, mast cells and their mediators. The physiological role of the reaginic mechanism has been emphasised above and, at least in part, is concerned with defence against protozoan and metazoan parasites, most of which are now rarely experienced in the Western world, e.g. malaria, trypanosomiasis and schistosomiasis. Parasite killing by IgE plus monocytes or IgG plus eosinophils (the latter recruited following ECF-A release by IgE-sensitised mast cells) have both been identified in recent years. The itching, scratching, hypersecretion, sneezing, coughing and contraction of smooth muscle which follow mast cell degranulation are also likely to be of considerable value in effecting the physical removal of parasites and their vectors.

The process of civilisation has led to a progressive decline in parasite load, and the introduction of novel environments associated with warm houses, modern diets (including formula feeding of infants), high pollen exposure and the keeping of pets has led to frequent contact with antigens by inhalation or ingestion. This process has been associated with a considerable reduction in the

**Table 11.3**   Atopic diseases.

---

Extrinsic allergic asthma
Allergic rhinitis
Atopic dermatitis
Allergic gastroenteropathy
Seasonal nephrotic syndrome

---

total and parasite-specific levels of IgE and thus the Fc receptors on mast cells tend to become preoccupied with IgE molecules with specificity for environmental antigens which do not constitute a serious infective threat to the host organism.

Genetic factors play an important part in determining suscep-tibility to atopic disease and several studies have reported significant associations between immune responses to pollen antigens and the possession of certain HLA haplotypes, e.g. HLA A1, B8, DR3. Figure 11.4 summarises the possible locations for the primary abnormality or lesion in atopic disease. The restricted molecular weight range of atopic antigens (25 000−45 000) might suggest that abnormal mucosal permeability could be a factor but this now seems unlikely. IgA is the usual protective antibody at mucosal surfaces and several studies have show an increased prevalence of IgA deficiency in atopic individuals and their relatives. Other work indicates the presence of genes which regulate the levels of IgE

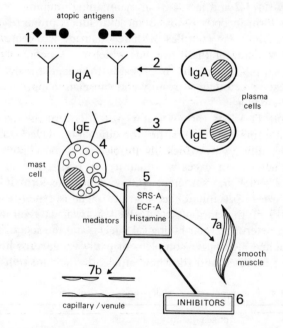

**Fig. 11.4** Possible locations of the primary abnormality in atopic disease: 1 — abnormal mucosal permeability, 2 — impaired IgA production, 3 — increased IgE production, 4 — inappropriate mast cell degranulation, 5 — variation in mediator production, 6 — deficiency of mediator inhibitors, and 7 (a and b) — abnormal susceptibility of target organs (e.g. smooth muscle and endothelium) to mediator effects.

production: a process in which suppressor T cells may have a role. Other possibilities concern the ease with which mast cells degranulate; qualitative and possibly quantitative variations in the mediators produced; abnormalities of other molecules which inhibit them (e.g. amine oxidase); and, lastly, variation in their effects on endothelial and smooth muscle cells. Earlier reports that the presence of antiglobulins reactive with IgE, i.e. anti-IgE, or antibodies reactive with β2 adrenergic receptors might be important have received little confirmation so far.

## Immune complex disease

It is interesting to speculate why some individuals should be particularly prone to the development of widespread immune complex disease following otherwise straightforward infections. Recently attention has focused on the role of complement components (particulary C4, C2 and factor B) in maintaining immune complexes in soluble form in body fluids. Some individuals prone to conditions in which immune complex-mediated damage is a feature possess genetic variants of these proteins which are functionally less efficient (see p. 73) and this is probably the major reason why their complexes precipitate so readily and cause an inappropriate degree of tissue damage.

Table 11.4 lists various factors which govern the deposition of immune complexes (IC) within the circulation. Overloading of the normal pathways by which IC are cleared is most likely to occur when there is an excessive quantity or persistence of antigenic material which has sufficient epitope density to form IC of a sufficient size to precipitate (see Fig. 5.8). The isotype (i.e. class and subclass) of the antibodies involved as well as their affinity of binding determine their biological effects, and the adequacy of both classical and alternative complement pathways governs how readily IC are solubilised and thus how efficiently they are transported to

**Table 11.4**  Factors governing the deposition of circulating immune complexes.

Antigen quantity and persistence
Antibody isotype and affinity
Solubilisation capacity of serum (C1, C4, C2)
Local factors
  Site of IC formation
  Turbulence
  Capillary permeability
  Filtration effects

cells of the mononuclear phagocyte series which are able to ingest and process them. Approximately 1 per cent of the population are heterozygotes for C2 deficiency and deficiencies of C1q, C1r, C4 and C2 are all associated with susceptibility to the development of immune complex disease (see Chapter 12).

The sites at which circulating IC are deposited will be determined partly by their site of formation, e.g. the release of large quantities of antigen from heart valve endothelium in bacterial endocarditis and its combination with circulating antibody give rise to considerable deposition downstream in the kidneys (and other organs which are major recipients of the arterial supply). Turbulence of blood flow and local increases in vascular permeability also affect localisation. A major factor determining the localisation of IC in the circulation is the various sites at which plasma colloid is filtered to produce other body fluids, e.g. renal glomeruli, choroid plexus, synovium, epidermal basement membrane and uveal tract. An aggregation/concentration effect occurs as soluble complexes pass across these semipermeable membranes and this is why the localisation of circulating IC may appear to be confined to a single location and in a subepithelial position, e.g. as in membranous glomerulonephritis.

Thus, the formation of soluble IC has an important physiological role and it is only when their formation or clearance becomes grossly disturbed that the manifestations of **immune complex disease** become of clinical concern.

# Further reading

Cohen S., Ward P.A. & McCluskey R.T. (1979) *Mechanisms of Immunopathology*. Wiley, New York.

Coombs R.R.A. & Gell P.G.H. (1975) Classification of allergic reactions responsible for clinical hypersensitivity and disease. In Gell P.G.H., Coombs R.R.A. & Lachmann P.J. eds. *Clinical Aspects of Immunology*, 3rd edn. Blackwell Scientific Publications, Oxford.

Haakenstad A.O. & Mannik M. (1977) The biology of immune complexes. In Talal N. ed. *Auto-immunity: Genetic, Immunologic, Virologic and Clinical Aspects*. Academic Press, New York.

Platts-Mills T.A.E. (1982) Type I or immediate hypersensitivity: hay fever and asthma. In Lachmann P.J. & Peters D.K. eds. *Clinical Aspects of Immunology*, 4th edn. Blackwell Scientific Publications, Oxford.

Reeves W.G. (1977) Atopic disorders. In Holborow E.J. & Reeves W.G. eds. *Immunology in Medicine*, 1st edn. Academic Press and Grune & Stratton, London and New York.

Wells J.V. & Nelson D.S. (1986) *Clinical Immunology Illustrated*. Williams and Wilkins, Baltimore.

# Chapter 12
# Immunodeficiency

The immune system and the complex inter-relationships of its components have evolved to cope with the enormous variety of pathogens which threaten the host organism. Individuals with congenital or acquired deficiencies of the immune system are much more prone to serious infection. These 'experiments of nature' have shed considerable light on the functional significance of the deficient components.

It used to be thought that clinical immunodeficiency was confined to a few rare and rapidly fatal disorders but some forms are quite common, e.g. deficiences of IgA or C2. Every practitioner should be aware of the major kinds of deficiency and ways in which they are diagnosed and managed. In the past they have often been missed and mismanaged.

## Important clues

A diagnosis of immunodeficiency should always be considered when an individual experiences infection unusually frequently, in unusual locations or with unusual organisms and it should always form part of the differential diagnosis in children who 'fail to thrive'. The organisms involved may be unremarkable but infections with opportunistic organisms, i.e. those that do not usually cause disease, e.g. *Candida* or *Pneumocystis*, should arouse suspicion that immunity is defective. An increased susceptibility to infection can, however, be due to various non-immunological abnormalities (Table 12.1) which are considered briefly in the next section. Figure 12.1 indicates the major sites of involvement of the immune system in the immunodeficiency disorders which are reviewed in this chapter.

### Non-immunological abnormalities

The skin and other epithelial surfaces of the body provide an important first line of defence against infection. Denuded areas of skin, e.g. in severe eczema or following burns, provide ready access for many organisms. Lysozyme is a bacteriostatic component of mucous secretions, and the acid pH of the skin, gastric juice and

126

**Table 12.1** Examples of non-immunological abnormalities associated with susceptibility to infection.

| Affected site | Disorder |
|---|---|
| Skin | Burns and trauma |
| | Eczema |
| | Hidradenitis suppurativa |
| Mucosa | Ciliary dyskinesia |
| | Cystic fibrosis |
| Impaired drainage of a duct or hollow viscus | e.g. bronchiectasis |
| Cofactor deficiencies | |
| Zinc | Acrodermatitis enteropathica |
| Iron | Mucocutaneous candidiasis (see p. 133) |
| Acid pH | Vaginal candidiasis |
| Cortisol | Addison's disease |
| Insulin | Diabetes mellitus |
| Vitamin B12 | Transcobalamin deficiency |

vaginal secretions normally inhibit the growth of many micro-organisms. Hidradenitis suppurativa is a dominantly inherited disorder in which an abnormality of the apocrine glands causes obstruction and infection in the axillary and inguinal regions and round the umbilicus and areola of the breast.

Kartagener's syndrome is a form of ciliary dyskinesia in which an intrinsic defect in ciliary function (absence of the ATPase containing dynein arms) causes defective mucociliary clearance with pulmonary, nasal and middle ear disease and impaired sperm motility. In cystic fibrosis, ciliary function is normal but impaired clearance is due to abnormalities of the mucus component. Impaired drainage of any duct or hollow viscus provokes infection whether it is due to congenital malformation or the damaging effects of infection itself, e.g. bronchiectasis.

Infection can follow alteration in the level of various other cofactors, e.g. zinc, iron and iron-binding proteins, vitamin B12, cortisol, insulin and interferon. The free iron level may be especially critical. The over-energetic treatment of the anaemia of infection with iron supplementation can exacerbate infection (many bacteria utilise iron), yet some patients with chronic candidiasis respond favourably to iron treatment. The levels of acute phase proteins (e.g. C-reactive protein) adapt to infective stimuli (via interleukin 1 release) but deficiency of these materials associates with tissue destruction without overt infection, e.g. $\alpha_1$-antitrypsin deficiency and pulmonary emphysema.

# Investigation of suspected immunodeficiency

It is often difficult to decide when some children are experiencing more than their fair share of infection, particularly of the upper and lower respiratory tracts, and a scoring system has been devised as a guide (Table 12.2). A score of 20 is regarded as the threshold for serious investigation and events in category C are virtually an absolute indication in their own right. The pattern of infection experienced by the patient often provides a useful clue to the nature of the underlying disorder (Table 12.3) and can simplify the process of investigation.

Initially, investigation should include a haemoglobin level, total and differential white cell count, platelet count, serum IgG, IgA, IgM, C3 and total haemolytic complement. A Schick test (to determine the anti-diphtheria response following previous immunisation) and measurement of isohaemagglutinins may also be of value. If these investigations are normal and a high index of suspicion remains, or if specific pointers are already identified, then more detailed investigation is indicated. This may include characterisation of T and B lymphocyte subpopulations, IgG subclasses, secretory IgA in saliva and phagocyte function studies. *In vivo* challenge with pneumococcal vaccine, tetanus toxoid or dinitrochlorobenzene may be useful in assessing the severity of a particular defect.

## Stem cell deficiency

This is the most severe defect of all and gives rise to **severe combined immunodeficiency** (SCID). It presents during the first few months of life with failure to thrive, persistent oral *Candida* infection, intractable diarrhoea and *Pneumocystis carinii* pneumonia. Infants often show a measles-like rash which may be due to a mild form of graft-versus-host disease following the transplacental passage of maternal lymphocytes. Maternal T cells have been identified in the circulation in some cases. Most patients have an eosinophilia but some lack other formed elements of the blood, e.g. leucocytes, because they have a defect which affects the myeloid stem cell as well (Fig. 12.1), a condition known as **reticular dysgenesis**. SCID infants may develop overwhelming infections with herpes and measles viruses, and inoculation with live vaccines, e.g. BCG or smallpox, is invariably fatal. Immunoglobulin levels are low and a proportion of cases have a homozygous deficiency of adenosine deaminase (ADA), which metabolises adenosine and deoxyadenosine. Heterozygote carriers for this deficiency can be identified and antenatal diagnosis of the homozygous deficiency is possible. Rare individuals with a SCID-like syndrome fail to express HLA glycoproteins on the surface of their lymphocytes – a condition known as the **bare lymphocyte syndrome**.

Patients with SCID succumb during the first few years of life unless their stem cell deficiency is rectified by bone marrow transplantation. This requires the identification of a suitable donor, accurate HLA matching of donor and recipient, and graft acceptance by the latter. A further problem is the frequent development of **graft-versus-host (GVH) disease,** the incidence and severity of which can now be reduced by 'laundering' the graft to remove T cells using monoclonal antibodies or lectin columns (see Chapter 14). The use of fetal liver, fetal thymus or cultured thymic epithelium as sources of stem cells has been less successful. GVH can even follow the transfusion of one unit of stored blood and the T

**Table 12.2**   A scoring system to assess the need for immunodeficiency screening in children (devised by Hosking & Roberton).

| Factor | Score |
|---|---|
| **A** | |
| Major infection, e.g. meningitis, osteomyelitis, pneumonia requiring hospitalisation | 8 |
| **B** | |
| Infection in preceding 12 months (score per episode): | |
| Severe colds[a] | 2 |
| Pharyngitis, tonsillitis, croup | 2 |
| Otitis media | 3 |
| Bronchitis or other chest infection not requiring hospital care | 3 |
| Superficial bacterial skin infection[b] | 4 |
| Staphylococcal abscesses | 6 |
| Persistent watery diarrhoea (under the age of one year) | 4 |
| Pyrexia of unknown origin | 2 |
| **C** | |
| Relative of a patient with immunodeficiency who genetically could have the same defect | 18 |
| Non-infective clinical features of classical immunodeficiency | 20 |
| *P. carinii* pneumonia unrelated to drugs | 20 |
| Lymphopenia ($<1000$ lymphocytes $\mu l^{-1}$) unrelated to drugs | 20 |

[a] Defined as sore throat, rhinitis, fever, alteration of activity (e.g. missed school).
[b] e.g. impetigo.

**Table 12.3**  Patterns of infection in selected immunodeficiency disorders.

| Deficiency | Example | Pattern of infection |
| --- | --- | --- |
| Stem cell | SCID[a] | Viruses, fungi and bacteria |
| T cell | DiGeorge | Budding viruses, *Candida*, *Pneumocystis* |
| B cell | Hypogamma-globulinaemia | Pyogenic bacteria |
| Spleen | Splenectomy | Pneumococci, meningococci and *H. influenzae* |
| Phagocyte | CGD[b] | Catalase-positive organisms e.g. staphylococci and *E. coli* |
| Complement | C3 | Pyogenic bacteria |
| Complement | C5, 6, 7, 8, or 9 | *Neisseria* e.g. gonococci and meningococci |

[a] SCID — severe combined immunodeficiency.  [b] CGD — chronic granulomatous disease.

cells contained therein require elimination by irradiation before transfusion to any patient who has defective cell-mediated immunity.

## Thymic hypoplasia

Between the sixth and eighth week of fetal life, the third and fourth pharyngeal arches give rise to the thymus, parathyroid glands, great blood vessels and part of the face and jaw. In the **DiGeorge syndrome** their development is arrested, with the result that affected individuals lack a thymus (or have a few small fragments elsewhere in the neck), have hypoplastic parathyroid glands and abnormalities of their great vessels, e.g. transposition or Fallot's tetralogy, and may show facial abnormalities, e.g. low set ears, small jaw and a short philtrum.

Medical attention is usually sought because of their congenital heart disease or the hypocalcaemia due to parathormone deficiency but the triad of *Candida* infection, *Pneumocystis* pneumonia and persistent diarrhoea is soon evident. The absence of a thymic shadow on chest X-ray can be a useful pointer if thymic involution has not already occurred due to age or illness. The severity of the T cell defect is variable: most cases have a few T cells detectable in blood, and B cells and immunoglobulin levels are often normal. These individuals are less prone to develop GVH following blood transfusion and this is in keeping with their incomplete T cell defect. The immunological abnormality can be corrected by grafts of fetal thymus or the administration of thymic humoral factors.

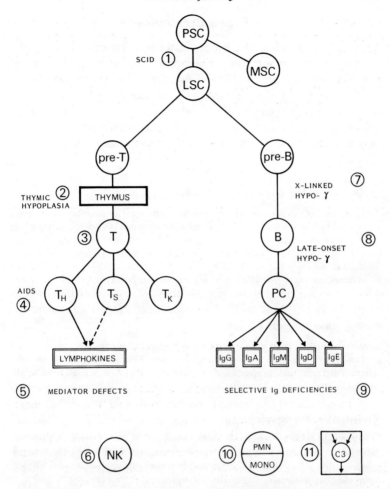

**Fig. 12.1** Major sites of involvement in **immunodeficiency disorders**: 1 — severe combined immunodeficiency, 2 — thymic hypoplasia, 3 — T cell deficiencies, 4 — acquired immunodeficiency syndrome, 5 — mediator defects, 6 — NK cell defects, 7 — X-linked hypogammaglobulinaemia, 8 — late-onset hypogammaglobulinaemia, 9 — selective immunoglobulin deficiencies, 10 — phagocyte defects, and 11 — complement deficiencies. PSC = pluripotential stem cell, MSC = myeloid stem cell and LSC = lymphoid stem cell.

Partial forms of the DiGeorge syndrome are not uncommon and, if the cardiovascular abnormalities permit and the hypocalcaemia can be controlled by the administration of vitamin D and calcium supplements, the infants usually show a progressive increase in T cell numbers and function with age.

# T cell deficiency

Various T cell defects have been described without evidence of a primary thymic abnormality. Five are referred to here, followed by the notorious acquired immunodeficiency syndrome (AIDS) (Table 12.4). T cell function can become abnormal for many other reasons, e.g. zinc deficiency (in acrodermatitis enteropathica), when lymphocytotoxins are present (as in various auto-immune diseases), and in many forms of secondary immunodeficiency (see p. 147 and Table 12.10).

### Purine nucleoside phosphorylase (PNP) deficiency

This, like the DiGeorge syndrome, is characterised by low T cell numbers with normal B cells and immunoglobulins but, in contrast, shows progressive deterioration rather than gradual improvement in immune status. These children are particularly susceptible to opportunistic viral infection and live vaccines can prove fatal. PNP is involved in the same purine salvage pathway as ADA and its deficiency is inherited as an autosomal recessive. There is, at present, no satisfactory way of rectifying this defect.

### Cartilage–hair hypoplasia

Some individuals present with abnormal T cell function, sparse thin hair, increased joint mobility and a form of short-limbed dwarfism. They are particularly prone to varicella infection, malabsorption and, in some instances, recurrent bacterial infection due to an associated neutropenia.

### Wiskott–Aldrich syndrome

This X-linked disorder consists of severe eczema, thrombocytopenia and susceptibility to opportunistic infection and usually manifests itself during the first few months of life. Most children succumb to infection although intracranial haemorrhage and lymphomas also occur. Affected individuals show a progressive decline in T cell function with profound lymphopenia developing by the age of six years. The

**Table 12.4**  T cell deficiencies.

Thymic hypoplasia (DiGeorge)
Purine nucleoside phosphorylase deficiency
Cartilage–hair hypoplasia
Wiskott–Aldrich syndrome
Ataxia telangiectasia
Chronic mucocutaneous candidiasis
Acquired immunodeficiency syndrome (AIDS)

serum shows decreased IgM, increased IgA and IgE and normal IgG levels and an absence of antibodies reactive with polysaccharide antigens including blood group isohaemagglutinins. IgG or IgM monoclonal proteins are occasionally present. All the features of this syndrome can be corrected by bone marrow transplantation. In the absence of an available matched donor, splenectomy is useful in reducing the risk of bleeding. The underlying abnormality consists of the absence of a sialoglyco-protein from the surface membrane of T cells and platelets.

### Ataxia telangiectasia

Cerebellar ataxia is first seen when affected children start to walk in their second year of life although the dilated small blood vessels (telangiectasia) do not usually become apparent until several years later. Repeated respiratory tract infection is usually complicated by bronchiectasis but lymphoma (often of T cell origin) is a common cause of death. T cells (and particularly helper T cells) are reduced in number and function whereas B cells are normal or increased. IgA is low or absent, IgE is reduced, IgG levels are usually normal and IgM levels are often raised. Auto-antibodies to IgA are often present. The condition is due to a DNA repair defect with increased susceptibility to form chromosomal breaks and translocations and is inherited as an autosomal recessive. Elevated levels of serum $\alpha$-1-fetoprotein and carcino-embryonic antigen are also related to abnormal gene control. No satisfactory treatment is yet available for this progressive disorder. The effect of irradiation damage on peripheral blood lymphocytes can be used as a diagnostic test and chromosomal radiosensitivity may permit the detection of carriers.

### Chronic mucocutaneous candidiasis (CMCC)

This is a heterogeneous group of disorders characterised by chronic infection of skin, mouth and nails with *Candida*. Most patients have normal serum immuno-globulins and very high levels of anti-*Candida* antibody. It is classified into four immunological subsets:

*Type I* with normal *in vitro* T cell proliferation but impaired macrophage migration inhibition factor (MIF) production.

*Type II* with impaired lymphocyte proliferation and normal MIF production.

*Type III* showing impairment of both lymphocyte proliferation and MIF production.

*Type IV* in which no immunological abnormality is detected apart from the presence of a *Candida*-specific inhibitory factor present in serum.

Most CMCC patients with normal specific immune responses to *Candida* respond to the administration of iron and folate and it is likely that iron deficiency is a key factor in the development of chronic candidiasis in many of these individuals. Some have associated endocrine abnormalities, e.g. hypoparathyroidism, adrenal insuf-ficiency and hypothyroidism.

# Acquired immunodeficiency syndrome (AIDS)

AIDS is a new and epidemic form of cellular immunodeficiency which was first recognised in young male homosexuals in the United States in 1979. It is also spread by promiscuous heterosexual activity and via infected blood and blood products, e.g. to intravenous drug users and haemophiliacs receiving factor VIII concentrates. Many cases have originated in Central Africa where its enteropathic form has become known as 'slim' disease. Affected individuals are prone to a variety of opportunistic infections, e.g. *Pneumocystis carinii* pneumonia, invasive perineal herpes simplex virus lesions and cytomegalovirus (CMV) pneumonitis (Table 12.5). An unusual feature is the prevalence of Kaposi's sarcoma (which is probably triggered by CMV infection and associates with HLA DR5 positivity), as well as various forms of lymphoma (some of which may be triggered by EB virus infection).

The causative agent was identified in 1984 and is currently, known as **human immunodeficiency virus** (HIV) (formerly called HTLV III or LAV). It is an RNA retrovirus possessing a reverse transcriptase which enables it to make DNA copies of itself within host cells. It parasitises T helper cells and the T4 molecule on their surface forms the specific receptor by which it obtains access to the cell. The human T lymphotropic virus type I (HTLV I) also infects the same lymphocyte subset but causes adult T cell leukaemia instead of inducing a cytopathic effect. There are interesting similarities between different members of the family of cell-transforming retroviruses and HIV may have arisen from a simian virus, e.g. STLV III, prevalent in Africa.

The immunological changes consist of a T cell lymphopenia mostly affecting T helper cells although impaired monocyte and natural killer cell function has been observed and impaired production of interleukin 2 and interferon is a usual feature. B cells and neutrophils are preserved and there are usually signs of polyclonal activation of B cells with hyperglobulinaemia and circulating immune complexes. Anergy to delayed hypersensitivity test antigens is a common finding.

AIDS is characterised by a latent period of between four months and four years (or more) between infection and development of the clinical disorder characterised by opportunistic infection and malignancy and, on present evidence, about 20–30 per cent of individuals exposed to HIV infection will proceed to develop AIDS. An intermediate form is known as **persistent generalised lymphadenopathy** (PGL). Serological tests for HIV antibodies are now available and it is hoped that a combination of rigorous public health measures and a reduction in sexual promiscuity will help to control the escalating incidence of this fatal disease.

Attempts to modify the course of AIDS by immunological

**Table 12.5**   The spectrum of infection in AIDS.

| Organism | Site of infection |
| --- | --- |
| *Candida albicans* | Oropharynx, oesophagus |
| Herpes simplex virus | Skin |
| Varicella/zoster virus | Skin |
| *Cryptosporidium* | Gut |
| *Pneumocystis carinii* | Lung |
| Cytomegalovirus | Gut, lung, retina |
| Mycobacteria | Gut, lung |
| *Salmonella* | Gut |
| *Toxoplasma gondii* | Central nervous system |
| *Cryptococcus neoformans* | Central nervous system |
| Epstein – Barr virus (EBV) | Mouth, lymphoid system |
| Human immunodeficiency virus (HIV) | Lymphoid system |

reconstitution — ranging from bone marrow transplantation to the administration of interleukin 2 and interferon — have been unsuccessful and most effort is being applied to the development of antiviral strategies, e.g. reverse transcriptase inhibitors, and the development of vaccines.

## Mediator defects

Lymphocytes produce a variety of soluble mediators or lymphokines and the chemical characterisation of some of them, e.g. interleukins and interferon, is well advanced. Impaired production of interleukin 2 is likely to be found whenever there is significant T cell deficiency but primary deficiencies of interleukins have yet to be described. Several reports point to the existence of patients who fail to produce interferon in response to viral infection and who are prone to develop fulminant hepatitis, herpes encephalitis or persistent EB virus infection. Defects of interferon production often go hand in hand with impaired natural killer cell activity and, in some instances, treatment with interferon has been shown to reverse an NK defect. Some children experiencing recurrent respiratory tract infection with rhinoviruses have deficient interferon responses and lack interferon in their nasal secretions. Deficient interferon production in leukaemia, systemic lupus and multiple sclerosis is likely to be a secondary phenomenon. Abnormalities of other lymphokines have been described, e.g. impaired production of macrophage migration inhibition factor (MIF) in recurrent herpes simplex infection (cold sores) and in some patients with chronic mucocutaneous candidiasis, but it is difficult to tell whether these abnormalities are primary or secondary.

## Natural killer cell defects

Natural killer (NK) cells, alias large granular lymphocytes (LGL), are particularly effective at lysing virus-infected cells, some tumour cells and cells of bone marrow origin (see Chapter 9) and are activated by all three varieties of interferon and by interleukin 2. Interferon deficiency can be associated with NK deficiency and restoration of the former can correct the latter.

Patients with the **Chediak–Higashi syndrome** are prone to bacterial infection and the development of lymphomas, and their cells show absent NK activity although the oxidative burst is preserved. Their leucocytes and platelets contain abnormally large and misshapen lysosomal granules and it is likely that the granule abnormality is directly linked to their NK deficiency. A similar condition has been described in mutant Beige mice. Impaired NK activity occurs in a subset of patients with late-onset hypogammaglobulinaemia in association with a high incidence of auto-immune disease. NK abnormalities have also been reported in fatal infectious mononucleosis and malignant lymphoproliferative disease and it seems likely that this deficiency impairs defences again EB virus and so permits the inactivation or transformation of B lymphocytes.

## B cell deficiency

An increased incidence of infection with pyogenic bacteria occurs with defects of antibody production or complement activation. This is because pus cells, i.e. neutrophil polymorphs, are the chief line of defence against these organisms and are recruited and activated following the interaction of specific antibody and complement. The major varieties of generalised antibody deficiency are described in this section (Table 12.6) Complement deficiencies are described on pp. 145–7.

## X-linked hypogammaglobulinaemia

In X-linked hypogammaglobulinaemia (**Bruton's disease**), affected males usually present with recurrent infection at between four

**Table 12.6**    Examples of primary and secondary hypogammaglobulinaemia.

| Primary | Secondary |
| --- | --- |
| X-linked (Bruton) | Myelomatosis |
| Late-onset (common variable) | Chronic lymphatic leukaemia |
| With thymoma | Protein-losing enteropathy |
| With dwarfism | Congenital rubella |
| Transcobalamin II deficiency | |
| Transient hypogammaglobulinaemia of infancy | |

months and two years of age. *H. influenzae, Str. pneumoniae* and staphylococci are the commonest organisms and the respiratory tract and skin the most frequent sites of infection. These children are protected from earlier infection because of the placental transfer of maternal IgG antibody. Episodes of diarrhoea may occur and are often due to infection with *Giardia lamblia*. A minority of patients develop arthritis which can be due to mycoplasma and responds to immunoglobulin replacement and chemotherapy. A few patients develop encephalitis (sometimes in association with dermato-myositis) due to an echovirus and although this can respond to vigorous immunoglobulin replacement it is often progressive. Other virus infections are not usually a problem although paralytic polio-myelitis can follow immunisation with the live attenuated vaccine.

The defect is one of inability of pre-B cells to differentiate into B cells (Fig. 12.1). Very few B cells or plasma cells are found in affected individuals whereas pre-B cells are present in normal numbers in bone marrow and show the typical absence of surface immuno-globulin in conjunction with the presence of cytoplasmic $\mu$ heavy chains. IgM and IgA are usually absent in serum and secretions and serum IgG levels are low but rarely completely absent. T cell numbers and function are usually normal. Although the disorder is X-linked, markers are not yet available for the identification of female carriers. In female infants presenting with generalised anti-body deficiency it is very much more likely that the underlying defect will be one of combined immunodeficiency with impaired T cell function. Male infants at risk should have their circulating B cell levels measured rather than wait for maternal antibody to decay so that replacement therapy can be started promptly.

A combination of immunoglobulin replacement therapy, rigorous use of antibacterial agents and measures designed to achieve maximal drainage of infected sites form the basis of the long-term management of generalised antibody deficiencies of all kinds. Immunoglobulin replacement has traditionally been administered by intramuscular injection at weekly intervals in a dose of 25–50 mg kg$^{-1}$ body-weight. Intravenous preparations are now available and usually need only be given at monthly intervals although they require close supervision and carry a risk of the transmission of hepatitis and other blood-borne viruses. The initiation of immunoglobulin replacement therapy can be as dramatically beneficial as the introduction of insulin therapy to the type I diabetic and, in both situations, careful follow-up is required for life.

## Late-onset hypogammaglobulinaemia

This is more common and much less consistent than the X-linked form and usually presents well after infancy and most often in the third decade. It is also referred to as **common variable** immunodeficiency. The pattern of infection is very similar and chiefly affects the lungs, sinuses and gastro-intestinal tract. Herpes zoster infection, meningitis, osteomyelitis and skin sepsis also occur. Some patients develop a form of malabsorption due to bowel infection with *Giardia*, *Campylobacter* or *Cryptosporidium*. Gastric atrophy and achlorhydria occur in about a third of patients and often associate with vitamin B12 deficiency although the typical auto-antibodies are not detectable and so a label of classical pernicious anaemia is debatable. There is also an increased incidence of gastric carcinoma, probably as a consequence of the achlorhydria.

Nodular lymphoid hyperplasia is often found in the gut. The nodules occur in the small bowel, resemble Peyer's patches and consist mostly of B lymphocytes. They are usually seen in patients with circulating B lymphocytes and preserved IgM production. Sarcoid-like granulomata are another feature of late-onset hypogammaglobulinaemia and are found in the lungs, liver, spleen and skin although no associated micro-organisms have been identified. Hepatosplenomegaly is the main clinical feature and this can be controlled with steroid therapy. Auto-immune haemolytic anaemia, thrombocytopenia and neutropenia are other complications seen in this group; these usually respond to steroids or may require a cytotoxic agent, e.g. vincristine.

Late-onset hypogammaglobulinaemia is often familial but there is no clear pattern of inheritance. Although the exact nature of the immunological defect is uncertain, cases divide into three main groups in which B cells fail to differentiate into plasma cells (Fig. 12.1):

1 Those with an intrinsic B cell defect.
2 Those with an immunoregulatory T cell imbalance.
3 Those with auto-antibodies to T or B lymphocytes.

In the first instance the B lymphocytes appear to be immature. In the second instance B lymphocytes are probably normal but fail to differentiate due to either a lack of helper T cells or overactivity of a suppressor T population. Some patients with late-onset disease have low NK activity.

Treatment is as for the X-linked deficiency, i.e. immunoglobulin replacement, antibacterial agents and drainage of infected sites with careful follow-up concerning the other complications to which these patients are prone.

## Other forms of hypogammaglobulinaemia (Table 12.6)

Patients with a thymoma often have an immunological disorder. Myasthenia gravis is the most common, with red cell aplasia and hypogammaglobulinaemia occuring in 10−20 per cent of cases. These patients lack pre-B and B cells. Excessive activity of their suppressor T cell population may be responsible for inactivation of the B cell series. Removal of the tumour can reverse the red cell aplasia but has no effect on the antibody deficiency.

Various kinds of dwarfism associate with isolated B cell deficiency and in one of these growth hormone deficiency is also present. Hypogammaglobulinaemia also occurs in an inherited deficiency of transcobalamin II, which can be reversed by giving large doses of vitamin B12.

**Transient hypogammaglobulinaemia of infancy** is probably underdiagnosed and occurs during the period when maternally derived IgG wanes and the infant's own antibody appears (IgM followed by IgG and IgA). The trough of antibody level usually occurs between the third and sixth months of life but can be more prolonged and is usually more severe in premature infants. Affected infants often develop troublesome infection; they have normal B cells but a relative lack of T helper cells. Some have immunodeficient relatives. The antibody deficiency usually resolves by the age of two years and immunoglobulin replacement is required until normal levels are attained.

Severe antibody deficiency can occur as a secondary phenomenon in a number of other diseases, e.g. protein-losing enteropathy (classically seen in intestinal lymphangiectasia), myelomatosis, chronic lymphocytic leukaemia and congenital rubella. Immunoglobulin replacement can be of value in addition to measures directed toward the primary abnormality.

# Selective immunoglobulin deficiencies

### IgG and IgA deficiency

These patients lack both IgG and IgA but show normal or elevated levels of IgM (and, in some instances, IgD). Plasmacytoid cells synthesising IgM (or IgD) are present in the circulation and in some tissues. The failure to produce IgG or IgA suggests an abnormality of the immunoglobulin heavy chain gene switch mechanism (see p. 59). Serum IgM levels and the associated lymphoid hyperplasia may decline when immunoglobulin replacement is given.

### IgA deficiency

IgA deficiency is one of the commonest forms of immunodeficiency, occurring in up to 1 in 200 of the general population. Most cases are sporadic but some have family members with varied forms of antibody deficiency. It has often been noted in patients treated with phenytoin or penicillamine, although the underlying susceptibility to develop IgA deficiency may be part of the primary disease for which they receive these treatments, i.e. epilepsy and rheumatoid arthritis, respectively. There is good evidence of an association between possession of the HLA A1, B8, DR3 haplotype and IgA deficiency. IgA deficiency is also a marked feature of ataxia telangiectasia (see p. 133). Patients lacking IgA are prone to sinopulmonary infection and bowel colonisation with *Giardia*, *Salmonella* and other enteric pathogens. Sporadic reports have pointed to a higher incidence of viral hepatitis, type I diabetes and other auto-immune disorders, and this susceptibility is probably due to defective handling of enteroviruses. Atopic disorders are also more common in IgA-deficient individuals (see p. 123).

Almost all IgA-deficient patients possess circulating B cells bearing surface IgA but these appear immature, often co-express IgM and fail to differentiate into IgA-secreting plasma cells. In some cases plasma cells producing the IgA2 subclass are present in the gut with the defect confined to IgA1-producing bone marrow plasma cells; in others, both subclasses are deficient. Circulating T cells which block the differentiation of IgA plasma cells have been identified in some patients with IgA deficiency.

Deficiencies in IgG2 and IgG4 isotypes, as well as IgE, are present in some patients with deficient IgA production. Examination of the immunoglobulin heavy chain gene sequence (see Chapter 5 and Fig. 5.7) indicates how these combined deficiencies might arise due to abnormalities of the immunoglobulin heavy chain gene switch mechanism or deletion of a section of the germ-line sequence. The latter possibility has been documented in a Tunisian individual found to be deficient in IgG1, IgA1, IgG2 and IgG4 who had normal levels of IgM, IgD, IgE and IgA2 with a raised level of IgG3. These variable associations may explain why only some individuals with IgA deficiency are prone to recurrent infection.

## IgG deficiency

Occasional patients are deficient in IgG but have preserved levels of IgM and IgA and these, as well as other individuals with normal total IgG levels but unexplained recurrent respiratory tract infections, often show abnormalities of one or more IgG subclasses. As mentioned above, defiencies of IgG2 and IgG4 can occur with IgA deficiency but lone IgG1 or IgG2 deficiency is also associated with recurrent infection. Antibodies reactive with some bacterial cell wall antigens are predominantly of the IgG2 isotype.

## IgM deficiency

Selective deficiency of this isotype is rare. Such patients lack iso-haemagglutinins and are particularly susceptible to meningitis and septicaemia with encapsulated organisms, e.g. pneumococci and meningococci.

## Immunoglobulin component deficiencies

Kappa chain, lambda chain and secretory component deficiencies have all been described in association with increased susceptibility to infection. In the latter case, neither IgA nor secretory component is detectable in saliva or jejunal fluid whereas the serum IgA level is normal. J chain deficiency has not yet been described but might be expected to give a selective abnormality with normal levels of monomeric IgG, IgA and IgM but absence of polymeric forms of IgA and IgM.

## Phagocyte defects

Phagocytes, i.e. neutrophil polymorphs and monocytes, have a critical role in defence against many bacterial pathogens. Profound neutropenia is associated with infection, septicaemia and ulceration of the mouth, skin and respiratory tract. Phagocyte function divides into three sequential components: (i) mobility, margination and adherence, (ii) phagocytosis, and (iii) intracellular killing (see Chapter 7). The primary phagocyte defects described below illustrate the importance of these different processes (Table 12.7). It is important to realise, however, that the presence of infection itself can cause secondary alterations in phagocyte performance. This may be due to toxic or inhibitory factors produced during infection or result from the recruitment of more mature cells, leaving earlier forms to predominate in the blood (often referred to as a 'left shift' in the segmentation pattern of neutrophil nuclei when viewing the blood film). In some families a cyclical neutropenia (with a periodicity of 3–4 weeks) can confuse the situation and serial studies may be required to identify this problem.

### Defects of mobility and phagocytosis

Various abnormalities have been described which affect the ability of phagocytes to migrate to sites of infection. This process involves margination and adherence to endothelial membranes, a directed response to chemotactic stimuli and adherence at the site of antibody combination and complement fixation. Immune adherence is

**Table 12.7** Primary phagocyte defects.

| Mobility ± phagocytosis | Killing |
|---|---|
| C3bi (CR3) receptor deficiency | Chronic granulomatous disease |
| Schwachman's syndrome | Myeloperoxidase deficiency |
| Actin dysfunction syndrome | G6PD deficiency |
| Absent specific granules | |
| Chediak–Higashi syndrome | |

intimately linked to phagocytosis and it is rare to find defects of phagocytosis alone. Not all mobility abnormalities are, however, associated with detectable abnormalities of phagocytosis.

These defects usually present with infections of the skin, mouth and respiratory tract but with little evidence of pus formation. Abscesses tend to be 'cold' and their pus 'thin'. Periodontal disease is common. Several disorders have been described, e.g. the **lazy leucocyte syndrome** and **Job's syndrome**, but there is considerable overlap between these clinical descriptions. Most of them are due to deficiency of a plasma membrane glycoprotein (of *c.* 150 000 MW) which is intimately related to the **C3bi receptor** (CR3). Affected individuals show impaired phagocyte mobility and complement-dependent phagocytosis but normal IgG-mediated phagocytosis and intracellular killing. Eczema and very high levels of IgE have been described in some cases but the link with atopic disease has probably been overemphasised. Delayed separation of the umbilical cord is a feature of some cases.

**Schwachman's syndrome**, in which neutropenia associates with exocrine pancreatic insufficiency and growth retardation, is another example of a neutrophil mobility defect due to a defective membrane protein. The **actin dysfunction syndrome** is due to the defective polymerisation of actin and decreased formation of microfilaments within the neutrophil. It gives rise to abnormalities of both mobility and phagocytosis. Cells from patients with the **Chediak–Higashi syndrome** also show defective mobility but with normal phagocytosis. They contain giant secondary lysosomes which contain the products of fusion of many cytoplasmic granules and the functional abnormalities observed may well be a consequence of the continuous activation which these cells undergo. They fail to kill catalase-positive and catalase-negative organisms and have absent NK activity although the oxidative burst is preserved, suggesting that the granule abnormality is directly linked to their NK deficiency. Some patients with recurrent infection and impaired neutrophil mobility have a **congenital absence of specific granules** but it is not clear whether the abnormality is due to lactoferrin deficiency or a reduction in receptors for chemotactic factors.

Phagocyte mobility is secondarily impaired in various disorders. The effect of infection has already been emphasised but impairment also occurs in malnutrition, burns, diabetes, uraemia and following the administration of various drugs and anaesthetic agents.

**Defects of intracellular killing**

The archetype is the rare but much studied disorder **chronic granulomatous disease** (CGD). Phagocytosis is normal but oxidative killing is absent in both neutrophils and monocytes. It is usually X-linked and affected male children develop infection — often taking the form of abscesses — of lungs, lymph nodes, liver and bones. Wound healing is slow and sinus formation may follow attempts at drainage. Other features include splenomegaly and gastro-intestinal involvement. It used to be called 'fatal granulomatous disease of childhood' but the outlook has improved with the advent of cell-penetrating antibacterial agents, e.g. trimethoprim and rifampicin, and an increasing number of patients are now surviving into reasonably healthy adulthood. The pattern of organ involvement is probably due to the uptake of neutrophils containing intracellular pathogens by fixed macrophages in bone marrow, liver, lungs and lymph nodes, where chronic granulomata develop and are difficult to eradicate.

The defect arises because of a failure to generate an effective membrane oxidase to initiate the oxidative burst which normally accompanies phagocytosis. CGD monocytes are also less efficient at antigen processing and presentation. There are probably several molecular causes of membrane oxidase deficiency, including an abnormality of cytochrome b involved in the electron transport chain linked to the membrane oxidase. Most of the problem organisms for patients with CGD are **catalase-positive**, i.e. they destroy any excess hydrogen peroxide they produce. Examples include many staphylococci, *Escherichia coli*, *Serratia marcescens*, *Salmonella*, *Aspergillus*, *Candida* and atypical mycobacteria. In contrast, organ-

**Table 12.8** Outcome of interaction between normal or CGD neutrophils and aerobic organisms (see text).

| Neutrophill | Microbe status | | Result |
|---|---|---|---|
| | $H_2O_2$ | Catalase | |
| Normal | + | + | Oxidative lysis |
| Normal | + | − | Oxidative lysis |
| CGD[a] | + | + | Microbial persistence |
| CGD[a] | + | − | Microbial suicide |

[a] CGD = chronic granulomatous disease.

isms which generate $H_2O_2$ and are catalase-negative, e.g. *H. influenzae* and streptococci, do not cause persistent infection. The reason for this disparity is that hydrogen peroxide produced in the absence of catalase can be incorporated into the metabolic pathway of the phagocyte to compensate for the lack of endogenous $H_2O_2$ production so that, in effect, the pathogen commits suicide (Table 12.8).

Several other enzyme deficiencies have been proposed as causes of defective phagocyte killing, e.g. deficiencies of myeloperoxidase and glucose-6-phosphate dehydrogenase (G6PD). In the former case the enzyme is deficient in neutrophils and monocytes although eosinophil peroxidase is preserved. Deficiency of either enzyme gives a clinical picture resembling CGD although the individuals are less incapacitated.

# Complement deficiency

Heritable deficiencies of each of the nine components of the classical pathway (including the three subunits of C1) as well a properdin and the inhibitors of C1 (C1 esterase inhibitor) and C3 (H and I) have been identified in man. Major deficiencies of C3 are associated with severe bacterial infection; deficiencies of components of the membrane attack pathway give increased susceptibility to infection with *Neisseria*, e.g. gonococci and meningococci; whereas deficiencies of early components in the classical pathway are associated with various forms of immune complex disease rather than overt infection (Table 12.9). Deficiency of the C1 esterase

**Table 12.9** Clinical associations of primary complement deficiencies.

| Component | Clinical picture |
|---|---|
| C1 esterase inhibitor | Hereditary angio-oedema<br>Immune complex disease |
| C1q, C1r, C1s<br>C4<br>C2 | Immune complex disease<br>    e.g. systemic lupus, vasculitis<br>    and glomerulonephritis |
| C3, factor I, factor H | Pyogenic infection |
| C5, C6, C7, C8, C9<br>Properdin | Gonococcal and meningococcal<br>    infection |

inhibitor is the cause of **hereditary angio-oedema**. Properdin apart, defects of alternative pathway components, e.g. factor B, have not yet been identified although the sera from some patients prone to staphylococcal infection and dermatitis have a defective opsonisation capacity which is likely to involve the alternative pathway generation of C3b.

Each of the deficiencies listed is inherited in autosomal recessive mode except for properdin deficiency, which is X-linked, and hereditary angio-oedema, which occurs as an autosomal dominant. C2 deficiency is the most common: approximately 1 per cent of the population are heterozygous for the deficient gene which occurs in linkage disequilibrium with HLA DR2 (see p. 48).

The biological products of C3 have a pre-eminent role in defence against pyogenic bacteria and the fact that only major deficiencies of C3 associate with severe infection emphasises the role of the alternative pathway in achieving C3 conversion when classical pathway components are deficient (see Chapter 6). Components of the membrane attack pathway only seem to be indispensable with regard to neisserial infections. The association of defects in the classical pathway with **immune complex disease** is a consequence of the role of these components in inhibiting the precipitation of immune complexes and facilitating their clearance from the circulation (see pp. 72 and 124). Deficiency of either of the two C3 control proteins (factor H — C3b binding protein — and factor I — the C3b inactivator) permits the unchecked activation of C3, leading to secondary C3 deficiency with a pattern of infection very similar to that found in primary C3 deficiency.

### Hereditary angio-oedema (HAO)

This condition usually presents by the age of 10 with episodes of subepithelial oedema of the skin, larynx or gastro-intestinal tract which last for 2–3 days. Oedema of the gut can present as severe abdominal pain and laryngeal oedema can prove fatal. C1 esterase inhibitor inactivates various serine esterases including plasmin, kallikrein, Hageman factor and factor XI as well as the activated forms of C1 (C$\overline{1}$r and C$\overline{1}$s). In its absence, C1 becomes readily cleaved (especially at extravascular sites where levels of another major enzyme inhibitor — $\alpha_2$-macroglobulin — are very low) with generation of the activated forms of C4 and C2 and, in particular, a vaso-active peptide derived from C2b by plasmin. This process does not cause effective C3 conversion as it mostly occurs in fluid phase without the generation of a stable membrane-bound C3 convertase (see Chapter 6). Thus these patients have low levels of C4 and C2 with normal C3.

The large majority of patients are heterozygous for C1 esterase inhibitor deficiency but their inhibitor levels are usually well below 50 per cent normal because of increased catabolism. A rarer form consists of heterozygosity for a dysfunctional form of the inhibitor. Patients with HAO also have an increased susceptibility to immune complex disease probably as a consequence of their secondary deficiencies of C2 and C4. The condition can be treated by giving inhibitors of fibrinolysis, e.g. ε-amino caproic acid and tranexamic acid, or the administration of androgenic steroids, e.g. danazol and stanozolol. The latter increase synthesis of the inhibitor and correct the C2 and C4 deficiency. Purified C1 esterase inhibitor is now available for replacement therapy by intravenous injection.

Acquired forms of C1 esterase inhibitor are usually associated with lymphoproliferative disease. This has been variously attributed to absorption of the inhibitor protein by tumour cells, the formation of anti-idiotype complexes or the presence of a monoclonal auto-antibody which inactivates the inhibitor.

# Secondary forms of immunodeficiency

The commonest cause of serious immunodeficiency in clinical practice is none of the above but rather the impact that a number of diseases and the therapies used to treat them have upon the immune system. Table 12.10 lists some of the more important examples. Depression of T cell responses occurs early on in Hodgkin's disease whereas antibody deficiency is usually a progressive feature of chronic lymphocytic leukaemia and myeloma. Other disorders associated with impaired protein intake or protein loss also cause immunodeficiency and secondary impairment develops during the course of most forms of chronic inflammatory disease.

## Lymphoid ablation

The surgical removal of tonsils, adenoids, appendix or local lymph nodes has little effect on immunological responsiveness although one should be reluctant to remove lymphoid tissue in individuals who already show signs of immunodeficiency. Removal of the spleen, however, greatly increases the risk of fulminant infection with pneumonococci, meningococci and *Haemophilus influenzae*.

**Table 12.10** Major causes of secondary immunodeficiency.

Leukaemia, e.g. CLL
Lymphoma, e.g. Hodgkin's disease
Myeloma
Malnutrition
Burns
Nephrotic syndrome
Protein-losing enteropathy
Uraemia
Down's syndrome
Chronic inflammatory disease
Persistent infection, e.g. malaria or leprosy
Congenital viral infection, e.g. rubella
Immunosuppressive drugs
Ablation of lymphoid tissue by surgery or irradiation

The risk is greatest in the first few years of life and within five years of splenectomy. Polyvalent pneumococcal vaccine should be given (and, where possible, before splenectomy is performed) in conjunction with prophylactic antibiotics. The immunological changes consist of impaired clearance of intravascular organisms, reduced concentrations of serum complement and IgM, and a disturbance of the normal profile of lymphocyte subpopulations, often with a moderate lymphocytosis.

Whole body irradiation with X-rays has powerful immunosuppressive effects, especially on the T cell compartment, and the technique of total lymphoid irradiation developed for the treatment of Hodgkin's disease has a profound and selective effect on T cell function. It has been used to facilitate graft acceptance and for the treatment of refractory auto-immune disease and appears to act as much by inducing suppression as by ablating help.

The use of powerful immunosuppressive drugs, e.g. corticosteroids, cytotoxic agents and anti-lymphocyte globulin, can also cause profound impairment of the immune system. The suppression of graft rejection in transplant recipients is still a balancing act between the development of serious infective complications due to generalised immunosuppression (particularly of T cell responses), on the one hand, and loss of the graft due to T cell-mediated rejection, on the other. The pattern of infection seen in these individuals is reminiscent of the problems experienced by individuals with primary T cell defects (see Table 12.3).

# Further reading

Hosking C.S. & Roberton D.M. (1981) The diagnostic approach to recurrent infections in childhood. *Clinics in Immunology and Allergy*, 1, 631–9.

Pinching, A.J. ed. (1986) AIDS and HIV infection. *Clinics in Immunology and Allergy*, 6, No. 3.

Rosen F.S. ed. (1985) Development immunology. *Clinics in Immunology and Allergy*, 5, No. 2.

Rosen F.S., Cooper M.D. & Wedgwood R.J.P. (1984) The primary immunodeficiencies. *New England Journal of Medicine*, 311, 235–42 and 300–10.

Soothill J.F., Hayward A.R. & Wood C.B.S. (1983) *Paediatric Immunology*. Blackwell Scientific Publications, Oxford.

# Chapter 13
# Lymphoproliferative disease

The study of lymphoid tissue was, until recently, a difficult task in view of the lack of clear and constant structural features and readily distinguishable cell types. Lymphocytes numerically overshadow the other cell types present in lymph nodes and recirculate through the lymphatic system. The delineation of the follicle-containing cortex from the medulla and the identification of specialised post-capillary venules (PCV) at their junction, started the process of understanding the relative roles and cellular constituents of these compartments and their cell traffic patterns (see Fig. 3.5). The development of antibody reagents specific for T and B lymphocytes and their subpopulations and the identification of various kinds of antigen-presenting dendritic cell, in conjunction with *in vivo* studies of lymphocyte traffic patterns, have led to an appreciation of the complex dynamics of lymphoid tissue and the way these processes are perturbed in disease.

## Lymphocytosis and lymphadenopathy

The common clinical problems are those of an excessive number of lymphocytes in the blood (**lymphocytosis**), enlarged lymph nodes (**lymphadenopathy**) or lymphocytic infiltration of other tissues. These can have many causes, including infection, auto-immune disease and neoplastic disorders. **Leukaemias** are characterised by the presence of abnormal white cells in blood and bone marrow. In **lymphomas** the normal structure of lymphoid tissues is replaced by abnormal cells of lymphoid origin and in some conditions, e.g. chronic lymphocytic leukaemia, both features coexist. Some forms of lymphoproliferative disease, e.g. **myeloma** and **macroglobulinaemia**, are associated with the production of excessive quantities of the secreted products of lymphocyte-derived cells.

The distinction between the characteristics of peripheral blood lymphocytes and lymphoid tissues (a) in the normal resting state, (b) during antigenic stimulation, and (c) in established lymphoproliferative disease has been greatly facilitated by the use of markers for normal, activated and transformed cell types. These markers include cytogenetic abnormalities; enzyme activities and polymorphisms; immunoglobulin isotypes (e.g. κ vs. λ); cell surface glycoproteins (e.g. HLA and various receptors); and, more recently, the ability to detect rearrangements in the genes coding for immunoglobulins and the T cell receptor proteins. This powerful armoury not only makes it possible to distinguish the cell type responsible for lymphocyte excess or infiltration but also enables the distinction to be made between proliferations which are **monoclonal**, i.e. derived from a single progenitor cell, and those that are **polyclonal**, i.e. derived from a variety of cells.

The three main categories of lymphoproliferative disease, i.e. leukaemias, lymphomas and monoclonal gammopathies, are now reviewed in turn. In each case, the abnormal proliferation of lymphoid or myeloid cells relates to a physiological counterpart and the particular stage of differentiation involved is indicated in Fig. 13.1.

## Viruses and oncogenes

The pathogenesis of lymphoproliferative diseases is poorly understood but the identification of several lymphotropic viruses, e.g. EBV, HTLV I, HIV (HTLV III) and the recently described human B lymphotropic virus (HBLV), in association with various kinds of lymphoma and leukaemia, suggests that infection with a virus belonging to this group may be a critical requirement. However, the very large majority of EB virus infections, for example, are self-limiting, due to an effective T cell response and it is probably only when this is deficient, e.g. in chronic malarial infection or in patients with AIDS or other forms of immunodeficiency, that B cell proliferation leads to overt lymphoma (see p. 159).

These cell-transforming or oncogenic RNA viruses contain **oncogenes** (V-onc) which, following the production of DNA transcripts (via reverse transcriptase), are able to alter the proliferative behaviour of the host cell because they code for growth factors, growth factor receptors or their second messengers, e.g. tyrosine kinases. The genome within human cells also contains similar sequences (C-onc) which are normally present in latent form (proto-oncogenes). These become activated in particular circumstances, e.g. during embryogenesis or clonal stimulation of lymphocytes. Several of the **chromosomal translocations** found in lymphoproliferative disease are known to affect the expression of host oncogenes, e.g. the transfer of material between chromosomes 8 and 14 in Burkitt's lymphoma and between chromosomes 9 and 22 which gives rise to the Philadelphia chromosome in chronic myeloid leukaemia. The relationship between infection with oncogenic viruses and the inappropriate expression of host oncogenes is currently an area of active investigation.

# Leukaemias

Leukaemia can develop slowly over a period of years or may present abruptly with clinical evidence of bone marrow involvement, e.g. anaemia, bleeding or infection. Leukaemia is designated 'acute' when more than 50 per cent of bone marrow cells are lymphoblasts or myeloblasts.

### Acute lymphoblastic leukaemia (ALL)

This is the commonest form of leukaemia in children. There are several types, which differ in the appearance of the leukaemic cells and their surface markers. The cells of the most prevalent form mirror the **lymphoid stem cell** (Fig. 13.1) in their possession of a surface glycoprotein — referred to as the **common ALL** (c-ALL) **antigen** — and their lack of both T and B lymphocyte markers (Table 13.1). The nucleus of these cells is also positive for the enzyme terminal deoxynucleotidyl transferase (TdT). Some cases are derived from pre-B cells and show cytoplasmic IgM with absent surface immunoglobulin and may be negative for c-ALL. Thymocyte or T cell-derived ALL shows positivity for thymocyte or T cell markers (e.g. CD1, CD2, CD3, CD5 — defined on p. 31) but is negative for c-ALL, HLA-DR and SIg (Table 13.1). B cell-

**Table 13.1** Cell markers in acute lymphoblastic leukaemia.

| | % of cases | TdT[a] | c-ALL[b] | DR[c] | Thy/T[d] | SIg[e] | Cμ[f] |
|---|---|---|---|---|---|---|---|
| Common ALL | 65% | + | + | + | − | − | − |
| Pre-B ALL | 15% | ± | ± | + | − | − | + |
| Thy/T ALL | 15% | + | − | − | + | − | − |
| B ALL | <5% | − | − | + | − | + | − |

[a] TdT — terminal deoxynucleotidyl transferase. [b] c-ALL — common ALL antigen, [c] DR — HLA DR. [d] Thy/T — thymocyte/T cell markers, e.g. CD1, 2, 3, 5 (see Table 3.1). [e] SIg — surface immunoglobulin. [f] Cμ — cytoplasmic μ chains.

derived ALL is the least common and is characterised by cells which possess surface immunoglobulin, are negative for TdT and often have cytoplasmic vacuoles.

Children with common ALL do well on a regimen of repeated courses of combination chemotherapy. Thy-ALL and B-ALL are more resistant to cytotoxic agents and have a tendency to relapse.

## Acute myeloblastic leukaemia (AML)

This occurs at all ages but is the commonest form of leukaemia in adults. It arises following the clonal proliferation of the **myeloid stem cell** (Fig. 13.1), normally the precursor of both monocytes and neutrophils. In AML the blasts usually show some evidence of differentiation to granulocytes, in contrast to ALL in which the blast cells show no differentiation at all. AML cells are positive for myeloperoxidase and non-specific esterase but are negative for TdT and the surface markers which characterise T and B cells and their precursors, including the c-ALL antigen.

Combination chemotherapy is used in AML but remission is more difficult to achieve and marrow failure is more difficult to reverse. Bone marrow transplantation is giving encouraging results in younger patients with AML in first remission although this option largely depends on the availability of a suitable donor.

## Chronic lymphocytic leukaemia (CLL)

This is a disease of the elderly, develops insidiously and can remain stable for many years. The circulating lymphocyte count may be 100 times normal and often without symptoms or physical signs. Younger patients have a more active course. Infection complicating secondary antibody deficiency and bone marrow failure are later sequels to which patients usually succumb. CLL does not transform into acute leukaemia but can develop into lymphoma.

The cell phenotype is that of the **mature B cell**, i.e. positive for surface immunoglobulin and HLA DR. In about 10 per cent of cases a monoclonal immunoglobulin is secreted of the same isotype as that detected on the surface of the CLL cells. Auto-immune haemolytic anaemia and auto-immune thrombocytopenia occur in a minority. Rare cases of CLL are of T cell phenotype and can be T4 or T8 positive. Cutaneous involvement is common and there is considerable overlap with the Sézary syndrome, mycosis fungoides and T cell lymphomas (see p. 157).

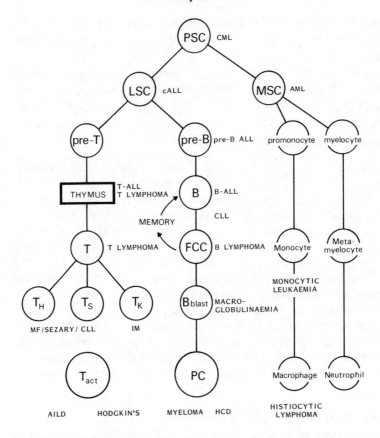

**Fig. 13.1** Differentiation pathways of lymphoid and myeloid cells, indicating the cell stages from which **lymphoproliferative diseases** arise. PSC — pluripotential stem cell, LSC — lymphoid stem cell, MSC — myeloid stem cell, FCC — follicle centre cell, $T_{act}$ — activated T cell, and PC — plasma cell. CML — chronic myeloid leukaemia, c-ALL — common acute lymphoblastic leukaemia, AML — acute myeloid leukaemia, MF — mycosis fungoides, CLL — chronic lymphocytic leukaemia, IM — infectious mononucleosis, AILD — angio-immunoblastic lymphadenopathy with dysproteinaemia, and HCD — heavy chain disease.

CLL is treated with prednisolone and/or an alkylating ágent when there is evidence of bone marrow failure, involvement of lymph nodes or spleen, or auto-immune haemolytic anaemia or thrombocytopenia. IM or IV γ-globulin is an important adjunct in those patients with secondary hypogammaglobulinaemia.

**Chronic myeloid leukaemia (CML)**

CML is a disease of middle life but usually presents with symptoms and signs of leukaemic infiltration, e.g. splenomegaly. The blood shows a marked increase in leucocytes (at least fivefold and often much higher). The abnormal cells derive from the **pluripotential stem cell** (Fig. 13.1) and show a cytogenetic abnormality — the **Philadelphia chromosome** — due to translocation of part of the long arm of chromosome 22 to the long arm of chromosome 9. Most patients develop a blast crisis in which the cell type transforms to give a picture resembling AML or ALL, underlining the common origin of the two cell types concerned.

Most patients with CML respond to treatment with an alkylating agent and splenic irradiation or splenectomy, where necessary. Bone marrow transplantation is being increasingly used in younger patients who have an HLA-matched sibling and this offers the prospect of long-standing remission.

# Lymphomas

In these forms of lymphoproliferative disease normal lymphoid tissue is replaced by abnormal cells of lymphoid origin.

## Hodgkin's disease

Hodgkin's disease typically presents in young adults with painless enlargement of regional lymph nodes. Histologically, it is characterised by the presence of large multinucleate cells of irregular shape known as **Reed–Sternberg cells**, which are surrounded by a mixed cellular infiltrate consisting of T and B lymphocytes, macrophages, neutrophils, eosinophils and plasma cells. Systemic symptoms such as fever, anorexia and weight loss are often present, particularly when lymph node involvement has progressed to other sites.

The origin of the Reed–Sternberg cell has been much debated and evidence has pointed in favour of both macrophage and T cell phenotypes. These cells are positive for HLA DR, may be positive for cytoplasmic immunoglobulin of *both* kappa and lambda type but are negative for surface Ig, suggesting secondary uptake of immunoglobulin. They often contain $\alpha_1$-antitrypsin but lack lysozyme, which is against a macrophage origin. Recent work with

Hodgkin's disease-derived cell lines and monoclonal antibodies raised against them suggests that these cells arise from activated T cells which are normally found in a perifollicular location and are positive for markers which are only present when T cells are in an activated state, e.g. the interleukin 2 receptor ($T_{ac}$). The inflammatory infiltrate and fever may thus be due to the persistent release of various lymphokines.

Hodgkin's disease is histologically classified into four subtypes: lymphocyte predominant, nodular sclerosis, mixed cellularity and lymphocyte depleted. Nodular sclerosis is distinct from the other three histological subtypes and is characterised by a nodular growth pattern which is encircled by collagen bands. Once this basic pattern is established it remains constant throughout the course of the disease. The subtype of Hodgkin's disease is important in predicting patient survival; those with lymphocyte predominant disease have the best survival and those with lymphocyte depletion the worst. Mixed cellularity and nodular sclerosis have an intermediate prognosis.

Treatment is dependent on the stage of the disease. If it is localised, radiotherapy is the treatment of choice but if further advanced, multiple agent systemic chemotherapy is used. Approximately three-quarters of patients treated for Hodgkin's disease survive for at least five years.

## Non-Hodgkin's lymphomas

The increase in our knowledge of the biology of the lymphocyte has led to a greater understanding of the commonest tumours of the immune system — the non-Hodgkin's lymphomas (NHL). This has given rise to more informative classifications of these neoplasms. The most widely used currently is the Kiel classification and the brief outline given here is based upon it. The majority (>90%) of non-Hodgkin's lymphomas are of the B lymphocyte lineage, 10% are of T cell origin and a small percentage express neither T nor B cell markers and are termed 'null' cells. The commonest forms of non-Hodgkin's lymphoma are derived from the germinal centre. In normal lymphoid tissue the germinal centre contains two kinds of **follicle centre cell** (FCC) which belong to the B lymphocyte pathway: the **centroblast** which is a large, nucleated cell with a rapid rate of division and the **centrocyte** which is a smaller cell with an irregular or 'cleaved' nucleus and a low mitotic rate. Neoplasms of the germinal centre are termed **centroblastic/centrocytic lymphomas** and in many cases recapitulate the architecture of the germinal centre and possess a follicular pattern. Less commonly centroblastic/centrocytic lymphomas may be partially or completely diffuse. Occasionally, tumours of germinal centres are composed exclusively of one cell type; either centrocytic or centroblastic. These lymphomas are always diffuse.

Malignancies of small lymphocytes are relatively common. They form a spectrum of disease ranging from cases with extensive marrow involvement, a peripheral blood lymphocytosis and inconspicuous lymphadenopathy to those whose clinical picture is dominated by lymph node involvement. The former picture is that of **chronic lymphocytic leukaemia** and the latter is termed **lymphocytic lymphoma**. The malignant cell appears identical in both processes and is a functionally immature B cell in the majority of cases. Lymphocytic lymphoma/B CLL is an indolent but incurable disease and many patients live for long periods, dying with the disease rather than as a direct result of it. A small percentage of lymphocytic lymphomas show evidence of early differentiation towards plasma cells. These are termed **lymphoplasmacytic lymphomas** and may be associated with the production of a monoclonal immunoglobulin. **Mycosis fungoides** is a cutaneous lymphocytic lymphoma of T helper phenotype which can spread to other organs. **Sézary's syndrome** is a related condition in which the skin changes are more diffuse and abnormal T cells are found in the circulation.

**Lymphoblastic lymphomas** are characterised by a proliferation of more primitive medium sized, nucleolated cells. Lymphoblastic lymphomas can be categorised into three main types: i.e. T cell, B cell and null cell. Many null cell lymphoblastic lymphomas express the common ALL antigen and are derived from pre-B cells. Lymphoblastic lymphomas have a poor prognosis and frequently become leukaemic. **Burkitt's lymphoma** is an unusual B lymphoblastic lymphoma which causes massive tumours in and around the jaw. It occurs in young African children who have had chronic malarial infection and is probably triggered by EB virus. It responds dramatically to chemotherapy. Post-thymic T cell lymphomas are relatively uncommon in this country (approximately 10% of all NHL) but are common in Japan and the Caribbean where they are associated with infection by the retrovirus HTLV I. The spectrum of T cell neoplasms appears at least as complex as B cell lymphomas but as a group they have a high frequency of cutaneous infiltration and hypercalcaemia.

Non-Hodgkin's lymphomas are treated with single or combination chemotherapy, with which some show long-term remission if not cure.

Enormous progress has been made in recent years toward disentangling the various forms and origins of lymphocytic leukaemia and lymphoma and the application of techniques derived from advances in molecular biology now provides the opportunity to detect the characteristic rearrangements of genes for immunoglobulins and T cell receptors found in stimulated cells of the B and T cell series. These advances are of particular value in ascribing cellular origins to that difficult residuum of lymphomas and leukaemias in which morphology and surface phenotype are unreliable. It will also help to distinguish monoclonal from polyclonal proliferations of the lymphoid system.

### Angio-immunoblastic lymphadenopathy with dysproteinaemia (AILD)

This condition is characterised by generalised lymphadenopathy, hepatosplenomegaly, skin rashes, fever and a polyclonal increase in serum IgG (and often IgA and IgM). Lymphoblastoid cells may be present in peripheral blood. The diagnosis is made on the basis of histological features in lymphoid tissue, i.e. a mixed cellular infiltrate containing immunoblasts, lymphocytes, plasma cells, eosinophils and histiocytes, marked proliferation of small blood vessels and deposition of an amorphous acidophilic material between the infiltrating cells. Anecdotal reports suggest that this condition may be triggered by various drugs, e.g. phenytoin or penicillin, or other antigens. A variety of autoantibodies are present and there is usually a haemolytic anaemia with a T cell lymphopenia and anergy on delayed hypersensitivity testing. Some cases spontaneously remit or respond to steroid treatment but 5–10 per cent of patients develop an immunoblastic lymphoma.

Recent work indicates that most cases show evidence of rearrangement of T cell receptor genes (without clonal rearrangment of immunoglobulin genes) suggestive of a monoclonal T cell proliferation. It is likely that the cellular infiltrate and blood vessel proliferation are the consequence of lymphokine release from the abnormal T cell population.

# Infectious mononucleosis

This condition is common and usually self-limiting but has interesting parallels and implications *vis-à-vis* other lymphoproliferative diseases. It occurs when primary infection with **EB virus** is delayed beyond childhood. The virus is spread by saliva and replicates in B lymphocytes. The transformation and proliferation of infected B cells is brought under control by T cells of cytotoxic/suppressor phenotype which recognise EB virus-determined antigens on the B cell surface. These immunological events coincide with the development of fever, sore throat, lymphadenopathy, splenomegaly and the appearance of **atypical mononuclear cells** (activated T cells) in peripheral blood. A variety of virus-specific antibodies can be detected as well as the typical heterophil antibody of the Paul—Bunnell test and some auto-antibodies, e.g. red cell and smooth muscle antibodies, occur transiently. After recovery, latently infected B cells are released into the circulation throughout life and are constantly eliminated by cytotoxic T cells.

The **Duncan** or **X-linked lymphoproliferative** (XLP) syndrome is a familial condition in which a defective T cell response fails to control primary EB virus infection, leading to uncontrolled B cell proliferation and the development of lymphoma. Nasopharyngeal carcinoma and Burkitt's lymphoma are also intimately linked to EB infection and a vaccine against EB virus is under active investigation.

## Monoclonal gammopathies

This is a group of disorders in which evidence of monoclonal proliferation is readily obtained due to the fact that the abnormal cells derive from terminal stages of the B cell maturation pathway (Fig. 13.1) and secrete large quantities of a chemically homogeneous immunoglobulin product. In **macroglobulinaemia**, the abnormal cell is a **B lymphoblast** which is found in lymph nodes, spleen and marrow and the secreted product is of class **IgM**. In **myeloma**, the abnormal cells resemble **plasma cells** and produce lesions in the marrow-containing bones without involvement of secondary lymphoid organs and the secreted immunoglobulins are of classes IgG, IgA, IgD or IgE. The organ distribution of the abnormal cells in macroglobulinaemia is in keeping with the presence of IgM-producing plasma cells in the medulla of lymph nodes and red pulp of the spleen but the localisation to the bone marrow of monoclonal plasma cells producing immunoglobulins of other isotypes is more difficult to explain unless these are cells which differentiate directly from pre-B cells in bone marrow or represent cells that have switched from IgM production and secondarily seeded in bone marrow.

## Macroglobulinaemia

Virtually all the symptoms of this condition are due to the presence of a **monoclonal IgM** of kappa or lambda type secreted by a population of cells infiltrating lymph nodes, spleen, liver and bone marrow which give the appearance of a slowly growing lymphoplasmacytoid lymphoma. The pentameric nature of secreted IgM (MW 1 million) leads to symptoms of blood **hyperviscosity** when levels exceed 30 g l$^{-1}$ and causes circulatory problems in the retina, central nervous system and extremities. Interaction of the monoclonal IgM with the surfaces of platelets, red cells and neutrophils may cause bleeding, anaemia and proneness to infection and in some cases the abnormal protein behaves as a **cryoglobulin**, giving rise to cold-induced peripheral vasospasm, i.e. **Raynaud's phenomenon.**

In contrast to myeloma, lytic bone lesions and the production of plentiful free light chains — Bence-Jones protein — are not features of this condition and thus bone pain, hypercalcaemia and renal failure are rarely seen. In contrast, rare cases of monoclonal monomeric (7S) IgM usually have the clinical features of myeloma (Table 13.2). Macroglobulinaemia is treated by plasmapheresis when hyperviscosity or cryoglobulinaemia is a problem in conjunction with drug therapy, which usually takes the form of prednisolone given with a cytotoxic agent.

# Myeloma

This is a malignant proliferation of plasma cells secreting a single immunoglobulin isotype of class **IgG, IgA, IgD, IgE** or **7S IgM** and containing light chains of kappa or lambda type. In about 20 per cent of cases the plasma cells secrete light chains in the absence of a heavy chain (Table 13.2). The abnormal plasma cells accumulate in bone marrow, replacing the normal marrow elements, and cause **bone pain** and, in some cases, pathological fracture (Table 13.3). There is an increased incidence of **infection** due to the development of secondary hypogammaglobulinaemia, neutropenia or interaction of the monoclonal immunoglobulin (if of isotypes IgG1 or IgG3)

**Table 13.2**  Incidence of monoclonal isotypes in myeloma.

| | |
|---|---|
| IgG | 55% |
| IgA | 20% |
| IgM[a] | 0·5% |
| IgD | 1·5% |
| IgE | 0·01% |
| Light chain only | 20% |

[a] This refers to monomeric 7S IgM. Monoclonal pentameric 19S IgM occurs in macroglobulinaemia.

with phagocytic cells . Decalcification of the surrounding bone and **hypercalcaemia** is due to the release of an **osteoclast activating factor** (OAF) from the myeloma cells. Patients often show a bleeding tendency due to interaction of the myeloma protein with platelets or coagulation factors. **Hyperviscosity** of the blood is less likely with increased levels of monomeric immunoglobulin but occurs when these approach 100 g $1^{-1}$ and is particularly marked with IgG3 proteins, which have a spontaneous tendency to polymerise. Some myeloma proteins also behave as **cryoglobulins**, giving rise to cold sensitivity phenomena.

Plasma cells normally synthesise an excess of **light chains** compared to their level of heavy chain production. Large quantities of monoclonal free light chain are produced in myeloma and this material, being of small molecular weight, passes readily into the urine. This feature was first recognised by Henry Bence-Jones in 1847 and has become known as **Bence-Jones protein**. These excessive amounts of light chain can, however, be toxic to renal tubules, and other factors, e.g. hypercalcaemia, hyperuricaemia, amyloid and dehydration, also contribute toward the development of **myeloma kidney**.

A **compact band** is usually present on zone electrophoresis of serum (see p. 49) but his can have causes other than a monoclonal gammopathy. Monoclonal immunoglobulins are identified by **immuno-electrophoresis** (see Figs 5.9 and 13.2) and a diagnosis of myeloma cannot be excluded until this has been performed on serum and urine. Some patients will only show a monoclonal immunoglobulin in serum whereas others with 'Bence-Jones only' myeloma will only show the presence of light chains in urine unless there is impaired filtration due to renal failure. In more severely affected cases the immunoglobulins belonging to other classes are reduced, probably related to marrow infiltration and suppression of normal plasma cells.

Abnormal plasma cells are usually apparent on conventional examination of a bone marrow sample obtained by aspiration or

**Table 13.3** Clinical features of myeloma at presentation.

| | |
|---|---|
| Anaemia | > 90% |
| Bone lesions | 80% |
| Infection | 50% |
| Hypercalcaemia | 45% |
| Renal failure | 45% |

trephine biopsy. Most patients show radiological evidence of bone destruction. Examination of bone marrow cells by immunofluorescence (see p. 64) is also useful in confirming the diagnosis of a monoclonal proliferation and in identifying the isotype.

The treatment of myeloma is unsatisfactory with only a modest increase in survival being obtained with cytotoxic drugs, prednisolone and measures directed at reducing the severity of renal impairment.

## Benign monoclonal gammopathy

Monoclonal immunoglobulins also occur in other conditions (Table 13.4) and some patients have monoclonal proteins which are either transient or persistent but of undetermined significance and not associated with malignant disease. This condition which has been called **benign monoclonal gammopathy**. This diagnosis is difficult to establish prospectively although patients who have a level of monoclonal immunoglobulin less than 20 g l$^{-1}$, have few (< 5 per cent) plasma cells in bone marrow, do not show suppression of other immunoglobulin classes, do have an excess of urinary light chains and lack bone lesions, show a much more benign course and may remain well for many years in contrast to the relatively poor outlook for most patients with myeloma. However, careful follow-up has revealed that about 20 per cent of such patients develop myeloma, macroglobulinaemia or amyloidosis within a ten year period.

### Heavy chain diseases

Rare patients have been identified who show excessive production of free heavy chains, e.g. the α chain of IgA, the γ chain of IgG, the μ chain of IgM and the δ chain of IgD. **Alpha chain disease** is the commonest of this group and is characterised by diffuse infiltration of the small gut with lymphoplasmacytoid cells secreting

**Table 13.4** Causes of monoclonal gammopathy.

| |
|---|
| Myeloma |
| Macroglobulinaemia |
| Non-Hodgkin's lymphoma |
| Chronic lymphocytic leukaemia |
| Primary cold agglutinin disease |
| Benign monoclonal gammopathy |

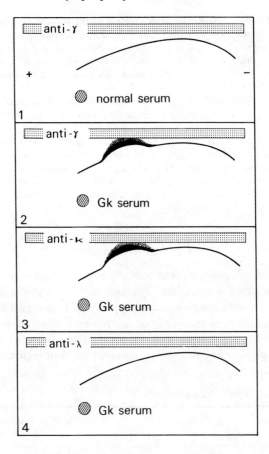

**Fig. 13.2 Immuno-electrophoresis** of (1) normal serum reacted with anti-gamma and (2, 3 and 4) a serum containing an IgG kappa monoclonal protein reacted with anti-gamma, anti-kappa and anti-lambda, respectively. Normal serum gives a long and heterogeneous line of IgG precipitation extending from close to the application well (⬤) to the cathodal end. The monoclonal IgG kappa protein gives a restricted 'bow' of precipitation (with the anti-gamma and anti-kappa reagents) which deviates from the normal IgG line and extends upwards toward the horizontal trough in which the anti-serum is placed. In myeloma and macroglobulinaemia, the amount of monoclonal protein may be so great that the precipitate redissolves in antigen excess (i.e. along its lower edge) and may merge with the antiserum trough. This can be overcome by examining the serum at greater dilution.

α chain dimers which usually show deletion of the variable (V$_{\mathrm{H}}$) region. Free α chains can be detected in serum by the technique of **immunoselection** in which the sample is electrophoresed through agarose-containing antisera reactive with kappa and lambda chains in order to precipitate all the intact immunoglobulin molecules, thus leaving any free heavy chains to react with an anti-α chain reagent in a second zone.

The incomplete nature of the abnormal immunoglobulin in this condition makes it difficult to ensure that this is a monoclonal abnormality. Some cases have remitted following oral treatment with antibiotics but most cases transform into an immunoblastic lymphoma of B cell type. Gamma chain disease behaves like a malignant lymphoma and γ chain fragments (often of the γ3 sub-class) can be detected in serum. Mu chain disease resembles chronic lymphocytic leukaemia with pentameric μ chain fragments present in serum and κ light chains in the urine, suggesting a monoclonal proliferation. A case of delta chain disease resembled myeloma but with free δ chains in the serum.

# Cryoglobulinaemia

The serum of some patients contains proteins which spontaneously precipitate or form gel-like polymers at temperatures below 37°C and are termed **cryoglobulins**. About 25 per cent of cases are due to the presence of **monoclonal** immunoglobulins (**type I**) which have an intrinsic tendency to cryoprecipitate (Table 13.5). **Type II** cryoglobulins are of mixed type (**monoclonal-polyclonal**) and con-

**Table 13.5** Types of cryoglobulinaemia

| Type | % of cases | Composition | Serum level | Diseases |
|------|-----------|-------------|-------------|----------|
| I | 25% | Monoclonal Ig IgM, IgG or IgA | 1–30 g l$^{-1}$ | Macroglobulinaemia Myeloma Lymphoma |
| II | 25% | Monoclonal–polyclonal Ig IgM–IgG IgG–IgG IgA–IgG | 1–5 g l$^{-1}$ | Macroglobulinaemia Lymphoma CLL[a] MEC[b] |
| III | 50% | Polyclonal–polyclonal Ig IgM–IgG | 0·1–1 g l$^{-1}$ | Systemic lupus Sjögren's disease Rheumatoid arthritis Vasculitis Chronic infection |

[a] CLL — chronic lymphocytic leukaemia. [b] MEC — mixed essential cryoglobulinaemia.

tain a monoclonal protein (most often of class IgM) with rheumatoid factor-like activity, i.e. it has specificity for IgG and forms complexes with it which tend to precipitate in the cold. This type of cryoglobulinaemia is associated with various kinds of lymphoproliferative disease including macroglobulinaemia. Overall, approximately 10 per cent of monoclonal IgM proteins have cryoglobulin activity: half of them spontaneously (type I) and half as a complex with IgG (type II). Some of the latter give rise to a clinical picture consisting of purpura, arthralgia, lymphadenopathy and hepatosplenomegaly in the absence of other primary disease — a condition known as **mixed essential cryoglobulinaemia** (MEC).

The remaining 50 per cent of patients with cryoglobulinaemia are of mixed polyclonal type (**type III — polyclonal-polyclonal**) in which polyclonal IgM rheumatoid factor-like antibodies complex with IgG and precipitate in the cold. These patients usually have an obvious immune complex disease, e.g. systemic lupus, rheumatoid arthritis or chronic infection, e.g. bacterial endocarditis. In each case the symptoms can be alleviated by plasmapheresis and the use of prednisolone and cytotoxic agents although treatment is directed against the primary disorder where possible.

# Amyloidosis

Virchoff gave the term **amyloid** or 'starch-like' to the material which can be deposited in tissue following chronic inflammation. These days this material is detected by the use of dyes such as Congo red or thioflavine t, by its birefringence under polarised light or by its fibrillary structure in electron microscopy. There are two main forms of amyloid. Light chain-associated amyloidosis is associated with lymphoproliferative disease and the excessive production of monoclonal free light chains. The main component of the amyloid fibrils is a protein, designated AL, which consists of light chains or fragments which include the $V_L$ domain. The other form of amyloid protein occurs in association with chronic stimulation of the immune system and is called amyloid A protein (AA). It has a circulating serum precursor (SAA) which is an acute phase protein similar to C-reactive protein. Both forms of amyloid also contain P-component which is identical to the serum amyloid P-component (SAP). P-component is not an acute phase protein but is present in the basement membranes of some tissues, e.g. the glomerulus. Prealbumin and some protein hormones can also adopt the typical fibrillar configuration of amyloid but these are numerically less important than the two forms described above.

## Further reading

Anon (1986) An unexpected new human virus. *Lancet*, **ii**, 1430–1.
Epstein M.A. & Achong B.G. (1977) Pathogenesis of infectious mononucleosis. *Lancet*, **ii**, 1270–3.
Gale R.P. & Hoffbrand A.V. eds (1986) Acute leukaemia. *Clinics in Haematology*, **15**, No. 3.
Habeshaw J.A. (1983) Lymphomas and leukaemias. In Holborow E.J. & Reeves W.G. eds. *Immunology in Medicine: a Comprehensive Guide to Clinical Immunology*, 2nd edn. Grune and Stratton, New York.
Jones D.B. & Wright D. eds (1987) *Lymphoproliferative Diseases*. MTP Press, Lancaster.
Kyle R.A. (1984) 'Benign' monoclonal gammopathy: a misnomer? *Journal of the American Medical Association*, **251**, 1849–54.
Lennert K. (1981) *Histopathology of non-Hodgkin's Lymphomas*. Springer-Verlag, Berlin.
O'Connor N.J.T. *et al.* (1985) Rearrangement of the T cell receptor β-chain gene in the diagnosis of lymphoproliferative disorders. *Lancet*, **i**, 1295–7.
Whicher J.T. (1983) Monoclonal proteins. In Holborow E.J. & Reeves W.G. eds. *Immunology in Medicine: a Comprehensive Guide to Clinical Immunology*, 2nd edn. Grune and Stratton, New York.

# Chapter 14
# Transplantation

## Histocompatibility systems

Vertebrates possess the ability to reject most cells or tissues obtained from sources other than those of their own genetic type and some invertebrates also display incompatibility reactions, e.g. genetically distinct corals growing on a reef. The speed and vigour with which tissues are rejected is related to their mutual degree of foreignness and the terms used to describe these differences are summarised in Fig. 14.1. Most of these inherited chemical differences belong to the **major histocompatibility system** (MHS) designated **H2** in the mouse and **HLA** in man and are described in more detail in Chapter 4. Other minor systems have a weaker influence on tissue compatibility. The genes of the MHS code for two kinds of cell surface glycoprotein: **class I** are present on all nucleated cells whereas **class II** glycoproteins are usually only present on cells involved in immune recognition, e.g. antigen-presenting cells, B cells and T helper cells (see pp. 45−48).

It has been estimated that at least 10 per cent of peripheral T

| RELATIONSHIP | NOUNS | ADJECTIVES | |
|---|---|---|---|
| 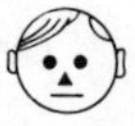 | Autograft | Syngeneic | Autologous |
| 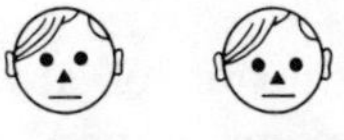 | Isograft | Syngeneic | Isologous |
| 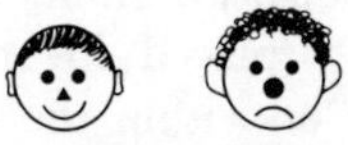 | Allograft | Allogeneic | Homologous |
| 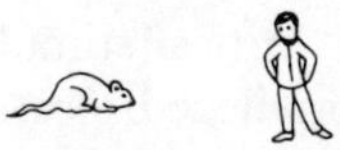 | Xenograft | Xenogeneic | Heterologous |

**Fig. 14.1** Terms used to describe immunological relationships.

cells can express reactivity to allo-antigens. This seemingly in-appropriate, if not eccentric, ability to react to foreign tissue specifi-cities does, however, have important physiological significance — implicit in the phenomenon of **dual recognition** (see p. 32 and Figs 3.2 and 3.3).

In essence, T lymphocytes — unlike B lymphocytes — recognise antigenic determinants conjointly with self HLA glycoproteins. T helper cells recognise antigen in association with class II glyco-protein on the surface of specialised antigen-presenting cells whereas T killer cells can recognise antigen in association with class I glycoprotein on the surface of any nucleated cell. This ensures that each subpopulation of T lymphocytes is guided to react with antigen in a functionally relevant situation. Recent studies with T cells specific for foreign antigens have demonstrated that such cells often show preferential binding for certain *allogeneic* histocompatibility glycoproteins, reinforcing the view that T cells see foreign tissues as 'self + x' (see pp. 29 and 34).

# The rejection process

The specificity and tempo of allograft rejection has already been illustrated in Fig. 1.2. Skin allografts continue to look normal for about 5 days after grafting but perivascular infiltration with lym-phocytes develops around day 7, followed by vascular obstruction and leakage with oedema and necrosis of the graft epithelium. Necrosis is usually complete by day 12 when the graft takes on a black and shrunken appearance. This process is accelerated if the recipient's lymphocytes have direct vascular access to the graft, e.g. as in a renal transplant.

## Afferent limb

For grafts which do not involve the construction of a vascular anastomosis, the process of recognition or 'sensitisation' usually requires intact lymphatic access, and grafts placed in specially constructed skin flaps or epithelial pouches or within the central nervous system may avoid rejection indefinitely: these locations have been referred to as **privileged sites**. The critical stimulus for the rejection of human tissues placed in unprivileged locations is the expression of class II HLA glycoproteins on the surface of antigen-presenting cells (Fig. 14.2). The T helper cell recognises foreign determinants in association with class II glycoproteins and

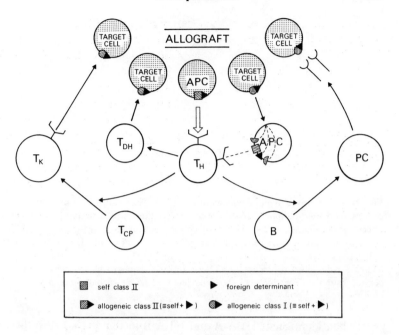

Fig. 14.2 **The induction of allograft rejection**. The presence of HLA class II bearing antigen-presenting cells (APC) within an allogeneic graft offers a direct stimulus to recipient T helper cells which recognise antigens in association with self class II. An alternative and less efficient route is for allo-antigens to be processed and presented by recipient APC, in which case only occasional processed fragments will produce effective stimulation.

The stimulated T helper cell then promotes (by release of IL2 and other lymphokines) the differentiation of killer T cells from cytotoxic precursors ($T_{cp}$) and plasma cells from B lymphocytes. T helper cells also release other lymphokines which attract and activate monocytes and these cells are referred to as 'delayed hypersensitivity' T cells ($T_{dh}$).

This diagrammatic summary uses the same symbols and conventions as Figs 3.2 and 3.3 (pp. 31 and 33) which also illustrate the phenomenon of dual recognition.

allogeneic HLA glycoproteins are recognised as a form of modified 'self'. Class I differences alone may not be sufficient to *induce* an allograft response. The necessity for class II differences to be present and that these should be expressed on intact cells is illustrated by the use of **mixed lymphocyte culture** (MLC) as an *in vitro* correlate of the afferent limb of the allograft response (Fig. 14.3). MLC relies on the ability of mixtures of mononuclear cells from non-identical individuals to stimulate each other in culture

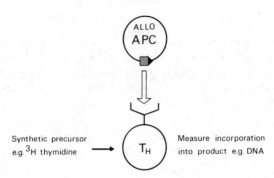

**Fig. 14.3 The mixed lymphocyte culture** (MLC). When allogeneic mononuclear cells purified from peripheral blood are set up in culture with a similar preparation of cells of self origin, the class II-bearing cells act as antigen-presenting cells (APC) and activate a proportion of the T helper cell population, i.e. the MLC mirrors the initial steps of allograft rejection as depicted in Fig. 14.2. This is quantified by adding a radio-labelled precursor of DNA, RNA or protein which becomes incorporated into these products as the cells increase synthesis and proceed to cell division.

even when identical at HLA-A and HLA-B loci and this led to the identification of the HLA-D locus, which is now more commonly characterised serologically by determining the equivalent HLA-DR specificities (see Chapter 4).

A major advance in recent years has been the realisation that much of the immunogenicity of grafted tissues is due to the presence of donor antigen-presenting cells — originally referred to as **passenger leucocytes** but now often called **dendritic cells** — which bear allogeneic class II molecules and present them directly to the recipient helper T cell without a requirement for intracellular processing (Fig. 14.2). Very few of these dendritic cells are required to elicit an allograft response and if they are removed prior to grafting so that induction of the allograft response has to occur via processing by recipient antigen-presenting cells then the response is very much weaker and less immunosuppressive therapy is required to prevent rejection. Only occasional processed fragments will resemble allogeneic class II (Fig. 14.2) and this route of sensitisation is very much less efficient than the direct presentation of allogeneic class II molecules by donor dendritic cells to which the helper T cells can respond directly. The relative immunogenicity of different allogeneic tissues follows the descending sequence of bone marrow, skin, pancreatic islets, heart, kidney and liver and largely relates to the quantity of class II-bearing cells within them.

**Efferent limb**

Once helper T cells become activated then the normal co-operative events (including the release of interleukin 2) enable killer T cells to differentiate from cytotoxic precursors ($T_{cp}$) with specificity for class I-bearing allogeneic cells and B cells to differentiate into plasma cells secreting antibody of allogeneic specificity. Graft rejection is also associated with the activation of monocytes which are probably induced by the presence of lymphokine-secreting T cells which differentiate directly from T helper cells and which have been designated 'delayed hypersensitivity' T cells ($T_{dh}$). The relationship between $T_{dh}$ cells and other T cell subpopulations is debated but killer T cells are not the only kind of T cell involved in graft rejection.

The response to an allograft transferred a second time — the 'second set' reaction — is more vigorous due to an expanded population of effector T cells which can operate without helper T cell stimulation. Specific antibody may also contribute to the more rapid rejection process. The balance between T cell and antibody-mediated effects varies according to the circumstance, e.g. the **acute rejection** of renal allografts is predominantly T cell-mediated whereas **chronic rejection** can be due to either or to a combination of both. In contrast, the dramatic events of **hyperacute rejection**, in which the kidney develops vascular stasis with platelet aggregation, neutrophil adherence and loss of function, are due to the presence of complement-fixing antibody in the recipient's circulation. This is usually avoided by a pre-transplant cross-matching procedure in which the recipient's serum is examined for the presence of antibody cytotoxic to donor cells.

# Ways of modifying the rejection process

Patients afflicted with end-stage organ failure are terminally ill or severely disabled, and when the kidneys are involved, face the prospect of regular dialysis for the rest of their lives. The realisation that patients in this category can be restored to a healthy and useful life following organ transplantation has given enormous momentum to the search for ways of ameliorating the normal allograft response (Table 14.1). Most of this knowledge has derived from work on kidney and bone marrow transplantation for, even now, the practicalities of heart, liver, lung and pancreas transplantation do not usually permit attempts at HLA matching.

**Table 14.1** Factors which help to modify the allograft response.

HLA typing and matching
Source and preparation of the graft
Selection and preparation of the recipient
Monitoring the allograft response
Non-specific immunosuppression
Specific immunosuppression
    (including the blood transfusion effect)

## HLA typing and matching

Typing of kidney donors and their recipients at the major class I loci — **HLA-A** and **HLA-B** — demonstrated that the degree of mismatch affected graft survival although the extreme polymorphism of these two loci means that it is relatively unusual to obtain a complete match between the four possible specificities of both donor and recipient. Incompatibility at the HLA-C locus seems to have little effect on graft survival. The introduction of **HLA-DR** typing by serological means indicated that matching for the rather smaller number of specificities at this class II locus had an even greater effect on graft survival in keeping with the pre-eminent role of class II glycoproteins in invoking the allograft response.

The procedures by which the limited supply of cadaveric organs is matched to the recipients' characteristics has reached an advanced state of organisation in many countries through agencies such as UK Transplant, Euro-Transplant and Scandia-Transplant. However, the urgent need of individual patients and the difficulties of finding perfect matches means that mismatched grafts are often used in renal transplantation. This is less feasible in bone marrow transplantation where the requirements are even more stringent (see below).

## Source and preparation of the graft

Most renal allografts are obtained from unrelated cadaveric donors and are often transported considerable distances in order to provide a satisfactory match between donor and recipient. The period of time during which the kidney is not perfused with an oxygenated blood supply (ischaemia time) is critical and should not exceed 45 minutes at 37°C or 24 hours at 4°C. For liver transplantation the cold ischaemia time is reduced to about 8 hours.

Living related donors are sometimes used in renal transplantation and in this situation it is possible to match entire haplotype (see Fig. 15.1, p. 188). The reduction in graft survival seen with one or two mismatches is such that some centres will only use kidneys from live donors that show matching of both haplotypes. However, the fact that about 10 per cent of such grafts fail within a year indicates the importance of other histocompatibility systems. Living donors are the normal source of bone marrow for transplantation and, where necessary, can be used on successive occasions.

There is particular interest, at present, in the possibility that pre-treatment of grafts with antibodies specific for class II-bearing dendritic cells linked to cytotoxic agents may render the graft considerably less immunogenic. Purging of bone marrow to remove T lymphocytes is now widely used as a means of reducing the incidence and severity of graft-versus-host disease and is discussed further on p. 181.

## Selection and preparation of the recipient

Many patients awaiting renal transplantation develop cytotoxic antibodies reactive with lymphocytes or endothelium following previous transfusion, grafting, pregnancy or infection. This state of pre-sensitisation to allogeneic tissue can lead to hyperacute rejection of a renal allograft and it is now routine procedure to perform a cytotoxic cross-match between the recipient's serum and the donor's lymphocytes. However, only antibodies with HLA-A and HLA-B specificity cause hyperacute rejection: HLA-DR antibodies are much less damaging and other autoreactive antibodies may even facilitate graft survival. It has been realised in recent years that the previously strict avoidance of blood transfusion to prevent pre-sensitisation operates to *increase* the chances of graft rejection and a standard protocol of pre-graft exposure to allogeneic blood is now standard practice in most renal transplant centres (see p. 178).

Another factor which confounds attempts to improve success by careful HLA typing and matching is that recipients who are positive for HLA-DRw6 experience worse graft survival than those who are negative for this specificity even when they and their donors are well matched at the DR locus. It is possible that this represents an immune response gene phenomenon (see p. 45). DRw6 also confers high responsiveness to *Streptococcus mutans*. An intriguing corollary is that the survival of DRw6-positive grafts is significantly better than those negative for this specificity, whether donors and recipients are well matched at the DR locus or not.

**Monitoring the allograft response**

Allograft rejection conjures up a dramatic picture of immunological events which should be eminently suitable to monitoring by the examination of peripheral blood for changes in antibody or lymphocyte characteristics. Many attempts, involving a wide range of antibody and lymphocyte assays, have failed to provide a clinically useful means of distinguishing rejection episodes from other events such as infection, or one that gives sufficient warning to be able to modify the outcome by therapeutic intervention. This may well be due to the fact that all the specific cells and antibodies of interest are preoccupied within the graft and thus not amenable to peripheral sampling.

A major advance, however, has been the recent introduction of **fine needle aspiration biopsy** of cells within renal grafts. Ten microlitre samples can be removed on alternate days without significant damage to the graft. The nature of the cellular infiltrate is a useful guide to the development of rejection and its severity: the presence of T and B cell blasts occurs early in the rejection process and infiltration with monocytes indicates severe and possibly irreversible change. It is interesting that a significant improvement in the survival of cardiac allografts — for which HLA matching is not attempted — followed the introduction of serial myocardial biopsy in order to observe the early histological changes of rejection. Otherwise, one is left with the non-immunological observation of graft function, using physical, biochemical, isotopic or electrocardiographic techniques which are very non-specific *vis-à-vis* rejection.

**Non-specific immunosuppression**

The potency of the anti-allograft response is such that none of the factors cited thus far are sufficient to achieve graft survival without the administration of drugs which suppress the immune system non-specifically. It is only following the exchange of grafts between identical twins (i.e. isografts) or when transferring tissue within the same individual (i.e. autografts) that immunosuppressive measures are unnecessary. In allotransplantation most rejection episodes occur during the first three months but a reduced level of immunosuppressive treatment is required indefinitely in the large majority of cases.

Most experience has been obtained with renal grafting and until relatively recently the standard regimen consisted of the antiproliferative drug, azathioprine (in a dose of *c.* 2.5 mg kg$^{-1}$ day$^{-1}$), in conjunction with the powerful anti-inflammatory corticosteroid, prednisolone, in a high dose of 100 mg day$^{-1}$ gradually reduced toward a maintenance level of 10 mg day$^{-1}$ at around 3 months. A controlled comparison of a lower dose (30 mg day$^{-1}$) of steroid given at the outset has demonstrated a similar effect on rejection and fewer side-effects and has replaced the high dose regimen in most centres.

All attempts at non-specific immunosuppression have side effects (Table 14.2), the most important of which is **opportunistic infection** followed by characteristic effects of the individual drugs used. The small but significant increase in the incidence of lymphomas and skin tumours is almost certainly due to impaired immunity to oncogenic viruses. Infection is still a major cause of

**Table 14.2** Side effects of non-specific immunosuppression.

**Infection**
    Viral, e.g. CMV, HSV, varicella/zoster virus
    Fungal, e.g..*Aspergillus, Candida, Pneumocystis*
    Bacterial, e.g. tuberculosis, *Listeria, Nocardia*

**Malignancy**
    Lymphomas
    Skin tumours

**Antiproliferative effects**
| Marrow suppression | Infertility[a] |
| Ulceration of GI tract | Hair loss[a] |
|  | Cystitis[a] |

**Teratogenesis**

**Steroid effects**
| Cushingoid appearance | Osteoporosis |
| Hypertension | Avascular bone necrosis |
| Diabetes | Cataracts |
| Peptic ulceration | Myopathy |
| Stunted growth | |

**Cyclosporin**
    Nephrotoxicity, hirsutism, gum hypertrophy

**ALG**
    Serum sickness

[a] Seen particularly with cyclophosphamide.

death in most transplantation programmes and emphasises the need for more sophisticated forms of immunosuppression. The subject of secondary immunodeficiency is discussed in more detail in Chapter 12.

The introduction of cyclosporin A has removed the necessity for continuous steroid administration and, in many centres, it is used as the sole immunosuppressive agent for renal transplantation. It is a fungal metabolite which acts specifically on T helper cells and is more effective than azathioprine in preventing rejection. This has led to further improvement in the one year graft survival figures for 1 and 2 DR mismatches (e.g. 81 per cent and 76 per cent), which now approach 0 mismatches which have survival figures of $c$. 85 per cent. It is used in a dose of around 10 mg $kg^{-1}$ $day^{-1}$ and is often reduced after 3 months although most centres titrate the dose to monitored blood levels of the drug in view of its variable absorption. The chief disadvantage is its tendency to cause nephrotoxicity but this can be largely avoided by blood level monitoring and dose adjustment.

Acute rejection episodes are treated with single shots of high dose corticosteroid (1 g methyl prednisolone intravenously or 200 mg prednisolone orally). The introduction of fine needle aspiration biopsy (see above) means that rejection can be diagnosed more accurately and maintenance doses of anti-rejection therapy, e.g. cyclosporin A, can be kept to a minimum with as few high doses of corticosteroid as necessary to deal with rejection episodes.

Many other forms of non-specific immunosuppression have been tried, including the administration of antisera (raised in various species) reactive with human lymphocytes and especially T cells. This material is called anti-lymphocyte serum (ALS) or anti-lymphocyte globulin (ALG) but as with every other approach to non-specific immunosuppression it has involved walking a tightrope between graft rejection and undue susceptibility to infection, often of an opportunistic kind. As ALS and ALG are of heterologous origin, patients sometimes show the features of serum sickness (see p. 102) on second or subsequent exposure.

### Specific immunosuppression

The prospect of inducing antigen-specific immunosuppression at will in the adult animal has been the goal of transplantation immunology since the 1950s when Medawar and his colleagues were able to induce a similar state in neonatal mice (Fig. 14.4). Experiment 1 demonstrates the normal rejection of a strain A skin graft

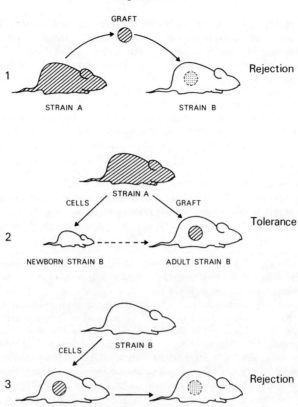

**Fig. 14.4** The induction of **immunological tolerance** in the mouse. Normally, skin grafts from strain A are rejected by the allogeneic strain B (experiment 1). However, if an animal of strain B is injected with cells from strain A when newborn it becomes tolerant to skin grafts from strain A for the rest of its life (experiment 2). This state of immunological tolerance can be broken by transferring lymphocytes from a strain B animal that has not been pre-treated to a tolerant mouse. This is followed by prompt rejection of the strain A graft (experiment 3). These experiments were first preformed by Billingham, Brent and Medawar (1956, *Nature*, **172**, 603−606.).

by a mouse of the allogeneic B strain. Experiment 2 shows that if cells from strain A mice are inoculated into newborn mice of strain B then the latter animals accept skin grafts derived from strain A throughout their adult life and have become specifically tolerant to this histocompatibility type. That the tolerant animals are immunologically normal apart from their specific unresponsiveness to allografts from strain A is demonstrated in experiment 3 in which the natural tendency to reject the strain A graft the animal already bears is restored by the infusion of cells from a strain B animal that has not been pre-treated with strain B cells when newborn. This effect is attainable in the mouse because of its immunological immaturity at birth and does not apply to most other mammals, including man.

Many other attempts have been made to induce immunological **tolerance** in adult animals and often with considerable success but the means by which graft acceptance has been achieved have not usually been clinically applicable or acceptable. It has been known for many years that the administration of graft-specific antibody can promote graft acceptance although there is always a risk of hyperacute rejection. This phenomenon of antibody-mediated **enhancement** has been studied extensively and, at one stage, received limited clinical application for renal transplantation. In experiments where prolonged graft acceptance has been achieved by this means it is clear that the initial phase of induction (or passive enhancement) achieved by antibody is replaced by a maintenance phase (of active enhancement) in which other mechanisms operate. Enhancement can also be actively induced by the administration of allogeneic cells or cell extracts prior to transplantation. These effects have usually been achieved across relatively minor transplantation barriers and only succeed in some donor–recipient combinations. When successful, the animals bearing enhanced grafts tend to show a progressive unresponsiveness to the donor strain. Some clinical examples have been recorded in which graft recipients have gradually 'adapted' to their allografts and been able to have most or all of their immunosuppressive drugs withdrawn.

Experimental studies have shown that the initial antibody-mediated phase of enhancement consists of the depletion of allogeneic class II-bearing cells from the graft. This may be achieved by a direct cytotoxic effect or may involve opsonisation by phagocytic cells. The maintenance phase of enhancement may be achieved by a process termed **antigen-reactive cell opsonisation** (ARCO) (Fig. 14.5) in which the continued production of allo-antibody forms complexes with alloantigen emanating from the graft, which act as a physical bridge between allo-antigen-reactive T or B cells and phagocytes which ingest (i.e. opsonise) the entire complex of antibody, antigen and antigen-reactive cell. This would explain the progressive loss of allo-antigen-reactive cells during the maintenance phase. Other experimental models support the proposal that the maintenance phase of enhancement is due to the progressive development of **T suppressor cells**. A third explanation concerns the development of **auto-anti-idiotype antibodies** (idiotypes and anti-idiotypes are described on p. 53). Experimentally, it has been possible to demonstrate that the injection of T lymphocytes bearing idiotypes specific for allogeneic specificities can induce anti-idiotype antibodies which will suppress allograft responses. However, it is usually necessary to inject idiotype-bearing cells or molecules in the presence of powerful adjuvants — a procedure which is not applicable to clinical transplantation. It is possible that suppressor cells which act to enhance graft acceptance may achieve this by expressing anti-idiotype activity and see below.

## The blood transfusion effect

The realisation that blood transfusion prior to allografting paradoxically increased graft survival has led to the routine inclusion of this procedure in renal transplantation programmes. The efficacy of donor-specific transfusions in living related kidney transplantation

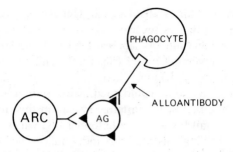

**Fig. 14.5 Antigen-reactive cell opsonisation**. If allo-antibody is present when allo-antigen (AG) is first released into the circulation of the graft recipient then complexes will form which, if they are not in antibody excess, are able to combine with antigen-reactive cells (ARC) of T or B cell type. This entire complex can then be internalised by phagocytic cells with effective loss of the antigen-reactive cell population.

could well be due to a specific effect akin to tolerance or enhancement. The fact that single random transfusions also have a beneficial effect in around 25 per cent of patients receiving unrelated cadaveric grafts is more difficult to explain although the appearance of suppressor cells with anti-idiotype specificity has been documented in animal models. Recent work suggests that *minor* histocompatibility determinants have an important role in the transfusion effect which may be mediated by specific or non-specific factors released from suppressor cells induced by transfusion. Between 1 and 2 units of blood is used clinically and can be given several weeks prior to grafting.

Total lymphoid irradiation (TLI) is another technique which can induce specific unresponsiveness and is currently under evaluation as a way of modifying responses in organ transplantation and auto-immune disease (see p. 148).

### Recurrent and transferred disease

Quite a few diseases leading to end-stage organ failure have an immunological pathogenesis and in these (as well as other conditions) it is possible that the original disease will recur in the transplanted organ. This problem is well documented in renal transplantation and the frequency of recurrence in dense deposit disease and focal glomerulosclerosis negates the value of transplantation. IgA nephropathy, Goodpasture's disease and Henoch–Schonlein purpura also recur but with less severity.

The transplantation of pancreatic islets is under investigation as a means of reversing type I (insulin-dependent) diabetes. However, a recent study demonstrated that specific destruction of the insulin-producing β cells could occur fairly soon after allografting, emphasising the role of the immune system in this disease. Cardiac allografts often fail because of atherosclerosis, which may resemble the patient's original disease, and individuals who receive a graft for congestive cardiomyopathy are particularly prone to develop a lymphoma. It is not unusual for leukaemia to recur in some patients treated with BMT but, rarely, the cells of the recurrent leukaemia have been shown to be of donor origin, suggesting transfection of an oncogene (see Chapter 13). Several examples of the transfer of atopic or auto-immune disease by BMT have been recorded.

The transfer of infection and malignancy are other possible hazards of organ grafting. In one case, a carcinoma developed following transfer of a kidney from a donor who was later found to have malignant disease. Fortunately, the tumour was rejected with the graft when immunosuppressive therapy was terminated.

## Bone marrow transplantation (BMT)

An advantage of bone marrow transplantation is that live donors are used and can be sources of marrow on successive occasions. A problem which is almost unique to BMT is that allograft reactions can occur in both directions, i.e. **graft-versus-host** (GVH) and **host-versus-graft** (HVG). This means that tissue matching has to be performed with greater accuracy, including mixed lymphocyte culture (for HLA-D specificities) as well as serological typing for HLA-A, B, C and DR. The permutations of the polymorphisms at these various loci are such that it is very unusual to find a satisfactory match from an unrelated donor and most marrow grafts are performed between siblings or parents and their offspring. The ideal situation, of course, is to have an identical twin. Marrow is aspirated from the iliac crests under local or general anaesthetic and is administered intravenously after passage through a wire mesh filter. The usual dose is *c.* $10^8$ marrow cells kg$^{-1}$ body-weight.

Graft acceptance is achieved by **conditioning treatment** of the recipient, which usually takes the form of cyclophosphamide with total body irradiation/total lymphoid irradiation/procarbazine or antilymphocyte/antithymocyte globulin given in addition. The risks of intensive irradiation are considered unacceptable in children, who usually receive a course of busulphan. This treatment means that the recipient shows severe deficiency of all blood cells (pancytopenia) for 2−4 weeks until engraftment takes place. Intensive support is required during this period in the form of red cell, white cell and platelet transfusions, intravenous feeding, anti-bacterial agents and a protected pathogen-free environment. The immune responsiveness of the recipient is severely depleted during the first few months and infection is a considerable hazard. Interstitial pneumonia due to *Pneumocystis carinii* or cytomegalovirus is a common problem and varicella/zoster virus infections are also a frequent occurrence.

### Graft-versus-host (GVH) disease

This complication might be expected to occur in all bone marrow transfers that are not syngeneic but is usually only obvious in 35−45 per cent of cases although it seriously affects the outcome. It is characterised by a diffuse rash, fever, abdominal pain and diarrhoea with disturbed liver function and, almost always, superadded infection. Its incidence is proportional to the degree of mismatch between donor and recipient and in recent years it has become customary to pre-treat the donor marrow with T cell-specific reagents in order to reduce the risk of GVH. This technique of marrow **purging** or **laundering** has improved the outlook for many patients and the reagents used have included complement-fixing monoclonal antibodies to human lymphocytes (and particularly T cells), lectins (e.g. soya bean) and immunotoxins specific for T cells. Clearly, these agents need to spare stem cells although how the subsequent differentiation of recipient-specific T cells from them is regulated is not clear. Possibly, such cells are brought under control by processes which survive the conditioning regimen and are comparable to the way in which T cell differentiation normally occurs in the thymus (see p. 28).

The introduction of cyclosporin A in the management of BMT has further reduced the incidence of GVH due to its preferential effect on helper T cells. However, in recent years it has become clear that there is a reciprocal relationship between the development of GVH and HVG responses in that a lower frequency of GVH associates with a higher incidence of graft rejection. The persisting problem of bone marrow graft rejection has led to trials of the administration of monoclonal antibodies specific for T cell subsets to the recipients and this has increased the incidence of engraftment, e.g. when reagents specific for both T4 and T8 cells are combined. There is also evidence to suggest that the responsiveness of T cells within the graft may be beneficial in patients who receive BMT for leukaemia, i.e. an anti-leukaemia effect, although the existence of leukaemia-specific antigens is still a matter of debate.

## Indications for BMT

The indication for BMT are the major immunodeficiencies, storage diseases and other inborn errors of metabolism, marrow aplasia and leukaemia (Table 14.3). BMT can be very successful in immunodeficiency and aplasia and the use of BMT to provide enzyme replacement for inborn errors is showing some promising results. BMT is starting to give encouraging results in patients with acute myeloid leukaemia (AML) in their first remission, for without such intervention most patients die from their leukaemia. However, the success rate with chemotherapy for acute lymphoblastic leukaemia (ALL) is so much better that BMT is usually retained for a sub-

**Table 14.3** Indications for bone marrow transplantation.

Immunodeficiency
  Severe combined immunodeficiency (SCID)
  Chronic granulomatous disease (CGD)
  Wiskott–Aldrich syndrome

Storage/metabolic defects
  Mucopolysaccharidoses, e.g. Hurler's disease
  Lipidoses, e.g. Gaucher's disease

Marrow deficiency
  Aplasia
  Agranulocytosis

Leukaemia
  Acute myeloid
  Chronic myeloid
  Acute lymphoblastic

Thalassaemia

Osteopetrosis

sequent relapse although it may be possible to identify the subset of patients who are prone to relapse so that they can be offered BMT early on. BMT is receiving increasing application in chronic myeloid leukaemia where elective intervention during the chronic phase is favoured before progression to blast crisis and this often produces cytogenetic remission with disappearance of the Philadelphia chromosome (see p. 155).

## Autologous transplantation

Some centres are adopting a more aggressive approach to certain haematological and solid tumours, in which the patient's marrow is stored before the patient is treated with intensive irradiation and/or chemotherapy, after which their marrow is returned. This also creates the opportunity to treat the marrow with anti-tumour antibodies and this has given encouraging results in ALL. However, it is too early to tell whether this will be useful in other forms of malignant disease.

# Further reading

Bishop G.A. *et al.* (1986) Diagnosis of renal allograft rejection by analysis of fine-needle aspiration biopsy specimens with immunostains and simple cytology. *Lancet*, ii, 645–50.

Brent L. & Batchelor J.R. (1982) The allograft reaction and its inhibition. In Lachman P.J. & Peters D.K. eds. *Clinical Aspects of Immunology*, 4th edn. Blackwell Scientific Publications, Oxford.

Catto G.R.D. ed. (1987) *Clinical Transplantation: Current Practice and Future Prospects*. MTP Press, Lancaster.

Fischer A. *et al.* (1986) Bone-marrow transplantation for immunodeficiency and osteopetrosis. *Lancet*, ii, 1080–4.

Goldman J.M. *et al.* (1986) Bone marrow transplantation for patients with chronic myeloid leukaemia. *New England Journal of Medicine*, **314**, 202–7.

Mason D.W. & Morris P.J. (1986) Effector mechanisms in allograft rejection. *Annual Review of Immunology*, **4**, 119–45.

Sutherland D.E.R. & Kendall D. (1986) Pancreatic transplantation: clinical aspects. *Diabetes Annual*, **2**, 94–119.

# Chapter 15
# HLA and disease

Initially, HLA typing was mainly performed to determine the degree of compatibility between donors and recipients prior to organ transplantation. However, it was soon realised that the presence of certain HLA antigens was positively associated with particular diseases (see Table 15.1). This chapter reviews the nature of this link between HLA and disease — a subject of considerable interest in recent years. The biological role of the HLA system and the structure of its proteins are dealt with in Chapter 4.

For many years serological typing (using a technique known as micro-lymphocytotoxicity) was only applicable to the **HLA-A** and **HLA-B** series of antigens and thus the first disease associations described were with these variants, e.g. ankylosing spondylitis (B27) and haemochromatosis (A3). Many other A and B antigen associations were described but when serological typing became possible for D locus antigens, i.e. **DR** typing, it was realised that many of these other diseases, e.g. type I diabetes, coeliac disease and rheumatoid arthritis, were more strongly associated with DR variants. The diseases listed in Table 15.1 are only a selection of those that have been described in the literature.

B locus associations are usually with diseases which are not of an immunological nature, whereas most of the conditions which are closely related to D locus variations are diseases in which immunological processes play an important part in their pathogenesis and this may give a clue to the underlying mechanism of association (see below). Some disorders, e.g. type I diabetes and coeliac disease, show association with more than one DR antigen and, in the former case, individuals heterozygous for the two antigens, i.e. who are DR3/DR4, are at greater risk than those homozygous for either DR3 or DR4, suggesting the presence of two different susceptibility genes or the formation of a novel heterodimer (see p. 48).

There are various ways of estimating the strength of these associations (see Table 15.1). A convenient way to display data obtained in a series of patients and controls with respect to the presence or absence of a particular antigen is in the form of a $2 \times 2$ table (Table 15.2). The **relative risk** (RR) is then the cross or odds

**Table 15.1** Associations between HLA types and some diseases.

| Disease | HLA type | Frequency (%) Patients | Frequency (%) Controls | Relative risk | Aetiological fraction |
|---|---|---|---|---|---|
| Idiopathic haemochromatosis | A3 | 76 | 28·2 | 8·2 | 0·67 |
| Congenital adrenal hyperplasia | B47 | 9 | 0·6 | 15·4 | 0·08 |
| Ankylosing spondylitis | B27 | 90 | 9·4 | 87·4 | 0·89 |
| Dermatitis herpetiformis | DR3 | 85 | 26·3 | 15·4 | 0·80 |
| Coeliac disease | DR3 | 79 | 26·3 | 10·8 | 0·72 |
| Sicca syndrome | DR3 | 78 | 26·3 | 9·7 | 0·70 |
| Graves' disease | DR3 | 56 | 26·3 | 3·7 | 0·42 |
| Type 1 diabetes | DR3 | 56 | 28·2 | 3·3 | 0·39 |
| Type 1 diabetes | DR4 | 75 | 32·2 | 6·4 | 0·63 |
| Systemic lupus | DR3 | 70 | 28·2 | 5·8 | 0·58 |
| Membranous nephropathy | DR3 | 75 | 20·0 | 12·0 | 0·69 |
| Multiple sclerosis | DR2 | 59 | 25·8 | 4·1 | 0·45 |
| Narcolepsy | DR2 | 100 | 21·5 | 135 | 1·0 |
| Goodpasture's syndrome | DR2 | 88 | 32·0 | 15·9 | 0·82 |
| Rheumatoid arthritis | DR4 | 50 | 19·4 | 4·2 | 0·38 |
| Hashimoto's thyroiditis | DR5 | 19 | 6·9 | 3·2 | 0·13 |
| Pernicious anaemia | DR5 | 25 | 5·8 | 5·4 | 0·20 |

Source: modified from Sveigaard *et al.* 1983.

**Table 15.2** A 2 × 2 table to display data concerning a possible association between the presence of an HLA antigen and the presence or absence of a disease (see text).

| | Number of individuals | |
|---|---|---|
| | HLA antigen positive | HLA antigen negative |
| Patients | a | b |
| Controls | c | d |

ratio, i.e. a × d/b × c. This value indicates how many times more frequently the disease develops in individuals positive for this antigen compared to individuals who lack it. Another estimate is to compute the **aetiological** ('etiological') **fraction** (EF), i.e. how much a disease is directly due to the disease-associated factor under investigation. This value can only be used when the RR value is greater than 1 (i.e. for those individuals who have an increased risk) and is determined by the following calculation:

$$EF = \left( \frac{RR - 1}{RR} \right) \left( \frac{a}{a + b} \right).$$

Those associations having a greater relative risk usually also possess a greater aetiological fraction but this is not universally so, for, where a particular gene has a very low frequency in the healthy population and is present in only a minority of patients with the disease, the aetiological fraction will be disproportionately low. An example of this is the possession of B47, which confers a relative risk of congenital adrenal hyperplasia of 15.4, which in Table 15.1 can be seen to be the same as for the association between HLA-DR3 and dermatitis herpetiformis, whereas the aetiological fractions for these two associations are 0.08 and 0.80, respectively.

The strongest HLA–disease association discovered so far is that between DR2 and narcolepsy giving a relative risk of 135 and an aetiological fraction of 1.0. The magnitude of the latter strongly suggests that HLA-DR2 is intimately involved in the disease process and may be linked to a receptor or neurotransmitter defect.

## Phenotypes, genotypes and haplotypes

HLA typing is usually only performed at the HLA-A, B, C and DR loci. In the absence of a significant degree of consanguinity, each individual is likely to possess a different set of HLA genes on the paternal and maternal chromosomes. The total set is known as the **phenotype**, which can be rewritten as the **genotype** when sufficient other members of the family have been studied to identify which genes belong to which chromosomes (Fig. 15.1). The collection of particular antigens which are under the control of genes borne on a single chromosome is known as the **haplotype** (e.g. a, b, c or d in Fig. 15.1). HLA haplotypes can be written in even more detail, e.g. the haplotype A1/Cw7/B8/DR3 usually possesses the following alleles at the intervening complement loci: C2C, C4AQO, C4BB1 and BfS, so that this becomes (reading from left to right along the short arm of chromosome 6) DR3 — C2C — BfS — C4AQO — C4BB1 — B8 — Cw7 — A2. This is termed the **extended haplotype**. Even though each of these loci is very polymorphic and the loci on each chromosome bear one of many possible alleles, certain alleles at one locus, e.g. HLA-A, are much more often found in the same haplotype in conjunction with certain alleles at other loci, e.g. HLA-B. These non-random arrangements are a common occurrence within particular populations and this phenomenon is known as **linkage disequilibrium**. The genes that confer susceptibility for HLA-associated diseases are very likely to be genes which are as yet undetectable but in close proximity with the major HLA loci and in linkage disequilibrium with them.

### Mechanisms of association

Several proposals have been made to explain the association between HLA types and disease (Table 15.3). It is likely that there is an array of **immune response** (Ir) **genes** in close proximity to HLA-DR similar to those described in the I region of the mouse MHC (see p. 45). Evidence in support of this comes from studies of the immune response to ragweed antigen (associated with HLA-Dw2), insulin (associated with HLA-DR7) and streptococcal extracts and allografts (associated with HLA-Dw6). Others have favoured the existence of specific immune suppression (Is) genes. One of the most striking features of the human MHC is the presence of four loci coding for important complement components and the fact that several of the extended haplotypes known to associate with some of the DR-related diseases contain genes which code for functionally inadequate or absent proteins. Individuals bearing certain haplotypes are less able to clear immune complexes from the circulation

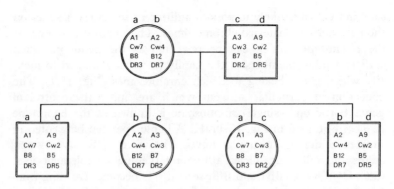

**Fig. 15.1** The inheritance of HLA haplotypes. See text.

**Table 15.3** Possible mechanisms of association of disease with HLA.

Immune response (Ir) or suppression (Is) genes
Complement or phagocyte polymorphisms
Molecular mimicry
Receptor interaction

and show significant differences in phagocyte function. It seems likely that variations in the quality of effector systems such as complement and phagocytic cells, i.e. **complement** or **phagocyte polymorphisms**, could be important in determining the outcome of virus infections which may damage host tissues whether an auto-immune response follows or not. It should not seem too surprising that class I and class II HLA glycoproteins, which have such a key role in lymphocyte recognition (see p. 46), should, when their bio-chemical type varies, have an effect in varying or modifying sus-ceptibility to immunologically mediated disease.

Others have argued that these disease associations occur because of chemical similarity, often called **molecular mimicry**, between the chemistry of these self proteins and chemical determinants present on invading micro-organisms. Most attention has been paid in this respect to the relationship between the possession of HLA-B27 and various 'reactive' arthritides, e.g. those which follow infection with organisms belonging to species of *Salmonella*, *Shigella* and *Yersinia*.

Evidence is also accumulating that HLA proteins may be inti-mately associated with hormone and virus receptors on the surface of cells, i.e. **receptor interaction**, and the extremely strong association between DR2 and narcolepsy may be an example of this.

## Contributions from other gene loci

Genes coding for structural variations in IgG molecules (the Gm system) and the acute phase protein α-1-antitrypsin (the Pi system) are both present on chromosome 14. These allotypic variations also influence susceptibility to a number of diseases and Gm and Pi alleles have an interactive effect with HLA alleles in various disorders, e.g. multiple sclerosis, myasthenia gravis and coeliac disease.

Recent developments in DNA technology involving the use of HLA gene probes and endonuclease restriction enzymes have enabled **restriction fragment length polymorphisms** (RFLP) to be identified within the HLA complex. More than 100 polymorphic sites have been identified so far and this approach will enable disease susceptibility or resistance genes to be mapped with greater accuracy and disease associations to be identified even when there is no evidence of association with any of the classical HLA polymorphisms. It should not be long before it will be possible to determine the identity of a number of HLA-related disease susceptibility genes and, more importantly, their likely site of action.

## Further reading

Bodmer W.F. (1984) The HLA system. In Albert E.D. *et al.* eds. *Histocompatibility Testing 1984*. Springer-Verlag, Berlin.

Reeves W.G. *et al.* (1984) HLA phenotype and insulin antibody production. *Clinical and Experimental Immunology*, 57, 443–8.

Svejgaard A., Platz P. & Ryder L.P. (1983) HLA and disease 1982 — a survey. *Immunological Reviews*, 70, 193–218.

# Index